Hey!
Who's Having
This Baby Anyway?

*How to take charge and
create a safe environment
for your baby's birth,
including essential information about
medications and interventions*

A Guide and Workbook

Hey!
Who's Having
This Baby Anyway?

*How to take charge and create a safe environment
for your baby's birth, including essential information
about medications and interventions*

A Guide and Workbook

*What Every Woman Must Know
About Childbirth*

Breck Hawk,
RN & Midwife

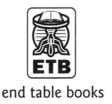

end table books

Copyright © 2005 by Breck Hawk

ISBN-10   0-9751264-4-X

ISBN-13   978-0-9751264-4-8

Library of Congress Control Number: 2004110432

CIP data

Hawk, Breck.

Hey! Who's Having This Baby Anyway? : How to take charge
and create a safe environment for your baby's birth, including
essential information about medications and interventions—a
guide and workbook.

/ by Breck Hawk.

p. cm.

Includes index.

1. Childbirth--Popular works.   I. Title.

RG652.H28 2005   618.4

QBI04-200353

END TABLE BOOKS

www.endtablebooks.com

email: *support@endtablebooks.com*

End Table Books is an imprint of *Metropolis Ink*
www.metropolisink.com

Cover design by Colin Hawk

DISCLAIMER

The opinions and suggestions expressed in this book are those of the author
and/or of their respective contributors. The author of this book is not a
physician. All decisions regarding your health and the health of your baby
should be made under proper medical supervision, therefore, the suggestions
contained in this book should not be, nor are they meant to be, substituted for
professional medical advice. You should consult a qualified physician before
you follow any suggestions in this book. The author and publisher disclaim
any liability arising, whether directly or indirectly, from the use and application
of any of the contents of this book.

Printed in the U.S.A.

Additional copies of *Hey! Who's Having This Baby Anyway?* may be
ordered directly from the publisher at EndTableBooks.com/HeyAnyway.

Queries about quantity discounts should be directed to the publisher at
Support@EndTableBooks.com

This is dedicated to:

My daughters, Farrah-Leigh and Rayna, because when they came into my life they became my world. They gave me the joy of being a mommy, and through them I learned what love really feels like.

To my mentors, Dr. Una Jean Sayles and Sandra Botting, who took me under their wings and taught me the art of midwifery. Thank you so much.

And especially to my very best friend in the world, Colin, who is also my partner and lover, and who supported me during the years of writing this with his patience, professional expertise and gentle criticisms. Remember, you may have loved me first, but I love you more.

ACKNOWLEDGEMENTS

To Barbara Harper for allowing me to use her article on Waterbirths. To Mickey Mongan for her constant support when I needed someone to vent to. To Tanja Johnson, my nurse manager at Three Rivers Hospital, for all the hugs, support and encouragement she has offered me. And to Cheryl Mokola for laboring over these words and making them flow nicely throughout the book.

And a special thanks to Kurt, Sandy and David for believing in this book.

Table of Contents

FOREWORD

By rights, books written for popular consumption should be an excellent source of education on childbirth, but here there's a real problem. I went to a large bookstore and surveyed the books offered on pregnancy and childbirth. There were twenty-eight such books, and twenty-three of them would have to be put in the category of obstetric party-line dogma, you know, the kind that insults the intelligence of women and urges, "Do what the doctor says, Dearie."

There is a simple test you can use to determine whether or not a book on maternity care is worth the reading. I call it the trust test. If the book says, "Ask your doctor," or "Trust your doctor," or "Listen to your doctor," it has failed the trust test and is highly suspicious and probably should go back on the shelf. If it says to trust yourself, trust your body, trust the scientific evidence, then you have probably come across something worth your while.

Hey! Who's Having This Baby Anyway? passes the trust test with flying colors. It is practical, sensible, honest, and completely respectful of you the mother and the family. The information is scientifically accurate and can be relied on. I strongly recommend it to every woman and family starting out to have their baby.

Professor Marsden Wagner, M.D., M.S.P.H., Perinatologist, Neonatologist, Perinatal Epidemiologist and former European Regional Office Director of the World Health Organization (WHO)

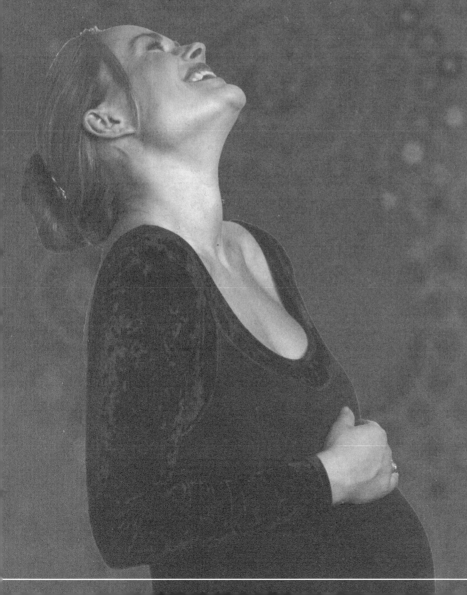

Introduction

Why this book?

Birth professionals—doctors, nurses, midwives, doulas, and others—have a remarkable variety of invaluable skills, ideas, and knowledge. But some of that information hasn't been readily available to prospective moms—until now. Oh, providers will give you the information if you ask, but unless you have the information in this book there are many critical issues they simply won't address.

This book will make it possible for moms to take charge and create a safe environment for their births, and it will tell moms about the risks and side effects of unnecessary medical interventions and drugs that are becoming so popular in the birthing industry. The information in this book will allow and encourage moms and dads to ask intelligent questions of their professionals, and to make informed, intelligent decisions based on their answers.

Beginnings

Twenty-eight years ago, when I was expecting for the first time, I knew nothing about pregnancy or having a baby. While I was growing up my mother didn't talk to me about periods or having children, or tell me what to expect on becoming a woman. I am the youngest in my family, so when I traveled right after graduating from high school I wasn't around when my brother and sister had their children. And when I did get pregnant I was living in Canada—hundreds of miles from my friends and family with no one familiar to talk to.

All of my life I had been pretty unconventional, and I wasn't going to handle my pregnancy and pending birth any differently. Against the advice of my friends and family, I chose to birth my baby at home. I didn't base my decision on what I had read or on extensive research, or even on discussions with other women; the decision came from the context of the lifestyle that I had been living for six years before my pregnancy. I was a product of the sixties (yea, Woodstock!) with its free way of thinking. Homebirth was a natural extension of that viewpoint.

I had excellent prenatal care. Dr. Una Jean Sayles, a Seventh Day Adventist and supporter of homebirths, cared for me throughout my pregnancy and the postpartum phase. Unfortunately, because of the Alberta Medical Association's political disposition at that time, this remarkable doctor lost her hospital privileges when she chose to practice homebirths. Canada in the seventies didn't support homebirths, and doctors in Alberta who attended births in parents' homes were forced by the Association to relinquish their hospital privileges.

My labor was a 27-hour ordeal. The time slowly ticked by, and I never had any idea what stage of labor I was in. We hadn't taken childbirth classes, so I had no clue about how I was supposed to breathe, what positions could help me, or how I could pace myself. No one knew how to help me through those painful and confusing hours, so for long periods of time I retreated to the bathtub or my garden. My partner didn't know what to do—those were the "no dads in the birth room" days, so most guys were pretty useless. Nevertheless, as in all births, there was no turning back, and after seeing the sun set twice and spending an hour and a half pushing, I gave birth to a pissed-off, pink and screaming baby girl. It was obvious that Farrah-Leigh wanted everyone in the room to know she had finally arrived.

In hindsight, I know my labor was long and difficult because I lacked both the knowledge and the warm, loving support women are designed to rely on during birth. I also know now how unrealistic it was to think that desire was all I needed to be successful at birthing.

A Midwife is Born

During the following weeks I became friends with Sandra Botting, a wonderful, warm, self-trained midwife who had assisted Dr. Sayles with Farrah-Leigh's birth. We spent hours together talking about homebirths in Calgary. Still flush from my successful homebirth and the fierce sense of pride it gave me, I wanted to help other women achieve what I had achieved. I wanted to teach classes, and I wanted to be there for pregnant parents when they had their babies, the way they wanted: at home, making their own choices.

Even though Dr. Sayles had lost her hospital privileges when she chose to do births at home, when she and Sandra asked if I'd be interested in helping them with homebirths in Calgary, still flush from the birth of my beautiful daughter at home, I said yes, and a whole new life opened to me, one that I still embrace twenty-eight years later.

I started my training by labor coaching and observing births with Dr. Sayles and Sandy. I gradually learned new skills, such as how to listen to fetal heart tones and check the cervix to monitor dilation. Eventually I was actually "catching" babies and placentas, doing well-baby checks, and helping moms with breastfeeding. We attended only about three to five births a month, and because of the Alberta Medical Association's policy against homebirth and its effect on the status of Dr. Sayles's license, Sandy and I had to be very careful with moms who had to be transported to the hospital. Parents in a transport situation had to either say that birth was precipitous or that they were birthing on their own. If it had been discovered that we were attending homebirths, the hospital would have reported us to the authorities.

Sandy and I studied for many long hours with Dr. Sayles. We immersed ourselves in our studies and tapped into every resource we could find about natural childbirth. We made *Williams Obstetrics* our bible. After a birth we would meet at her home or mine and talk about what we had seen, what we learned, and how to make the next birth better. We took a correspondence course from Suzanne Arms, the founder of the Association for Childbirth at Home, Intl. (ACHI), the very best prenatal classes for parents planning a homebirth. When we graduated we became ACHI instructors and proudly started a chapter in Calgary. We held fundraisers to help support other birth-related organizations. The more energy we contributed to homebirth the more we saw birth become easier, faster, and less prone to complications.

The Second Time's a Charm

Two years later, I was pregnant again. This time I had help; I was also well informed about the process of birth. My second daughter made her appearance in just two short hours. My body and mind knew every step, and I allowed myself to sail through each phase of labor. My inner knowledge and my circle of support guided me. I had no fear! The stages of labor flowed together, and my body birthed my baby without hesitation. This daughter was quiet and calm right after birth. She looked around the room, taking in everything. Her face was soft and showed no signs of distress or that her journey had been long or painful. We named her Rayna Duhna.

I continued teaching childbirth classes and attending homebirths for six more years before returning to the States. I loved everything about it— working with pregnant parents, helping moms birth their babies, and being involved in the community as it began to accept the idea of homebirth.

From Direct Entry Midwife (DEM) to RN

All was not as rosy in my personal life, however. My marriage deteriorated, and I was faced with being a single mom supporting my two daughters alone. I moved to Oregon with my girls and enrolled in nursing school, studying to become a certified nurse-midwife (CNM). The girls and I struggled to make ends meet.

When I received my associate degree in nursing and my license as a registered nurse I decided to take a position at the local hospital—I didn't have the heart, after so much struggle, to put my daughters through another two years of my being in school in order to receive my certified nurse midwifery license.

At first I thought I'd like to be a labor and delivery nurse, but after six years of attending homebirths I couldn't adjust to the hospital policies and procedures about birth or the ongoing—and what I felt were unsafe— medical interventions that providers were offering, or even insisting on, for their patients. So I took a position in the neonatal intensive care unit (NICU) where I worked with premature and sick infants who were less than six months old.

After eight years there, I was finally able to feel comfortable about nursing in the labor and delivery unit and worked there when the NICU was slow. After such a long time away from birthing, it was wonderful to be working with laboring moms and their families again.

Doula and The City

After my girls grew up, and 14 years after my divorce, I remarried and my husband and I moved to San Francisco. Colin's business as art director for an advertising agency became so successful we decided I could quit nursing in an institution and return to helping moms with their pregnancies and births. I started my own doula practice, "Doula and the City," and happily practiced as a birth and postpartum doula for two years.

I had never heard the term doula before we moved to San Francisco.

Women who helped other women in labor were usually called labor coaches or birth assistants. The job was the same—teaching, educating, assisting, and celebrating the birth of their children—but most were self-trained. Doula is a Greek word with many translations, but it essentially means a woman experienced in childbirth that provides continuous physical, emotional, and informative support to the mother before, during, and just after childbirth.

In other words, a doula is a birth professional that nurtures the woman and her partner throughout the prenatal period and through labor, birth, and postpartum days. She is an advocate for the mother-child dyad. Most doulas are not self-taught; they are professionally trained to be birth attendants in hospitals and homes. I met extraordinary and dedicated birth professionals in the Bay area. I listened to their amazing stories and shared my ideas about how to improve their birth experiences.

With the help of birth professionals and the support they give to laboring women, numerous studies have shown that the length of labor is shorter and presents fewer complications then a labor that is unassisted by a good support system.[1-3] For example, moms who have with them a birth professional during labor need far less oxytocin to augment labor, make fewer requests for pain medications or epidurals, and have fewer cesareans. The mother is much more satisfied with her birth experience, and she has less postpartum depression. Babies benefit too. They breastfeed more successfully, have shorter hospital stays, and they bond much more strongly with their mothers postpartum. As an added perk, the healthcare system benefits when moms use birth professionals because obstetrical care and hospital stays are reduced, which of course cuts healthcare costs.

The Times They Are a-Changin'

Sadly, medical institutions are losing their nurses, and they are desperately short staffed. Women don't have to be nurses and teachers anymore to earn a decent salary. Now they can be CEOs of large corporations, presidents of prosperous dot-com companies, or owners of big businesses. This turn of events has helped create a serious nursing shortage all across the United States and has all but eliminated the special one-on-one care that patients usually received in the past. When I was a floor nurse in 1988, I was responsible for four or five patients a night. Ten years later, floor nurses were often assigned to eight or nine patients. And it's getting worse all the time.

When I was working in a family birth center and in the NICU, I discovered that the work load in labor and delivery units is no different. In most cases, management of care has gone from one nurse for each laboring mom to one nurse for two to three laboring moms. Fewer nurses simply means less care for each patient, and the chance of one nurse continually staying with a laboring mom throughout her labor is rare—she'd probably like to do that, but she is just too busy. The sad truth is that if a nurse is to manage such a heavy load, she may rely on her pregnant patient's willingness to accept epidurals as pain management, allowing the mom to sleep while laboring, which could free her up for her other patients. But as you'll see later in this book, this method of management is not safe for mother or baby.[4]

I find that some pregnant women are easily manipulated and accept procedures while they're in labor simply to accommodate the provider and staffing situation. They're encouraged to give their okay for medical interventions to help speed up their labor and birth their babies in a timely manner. The use of epidurals and Pitocin or Cytotec (to induce labor) is becoming an accepted way—the standard way—of practicing medicine. Pregnant women are encouraged, with very little information beforehand, to welcome the chance to have their baby on a scheduled date for the convenience of their provider. Some even ask their providers to be induced for their family's own convenience. But they're often not told the risks and side effects involved for them and their baby. Pregnant women are blindly trusting their providers, thinking that everything suggested is for the good of them and their baby—but this isn't always the case.

Hey! Who's Having This Baby Anyway?

The information offered in this book must be made available to moms to inform them of their choices; to alert them as to what can happen because of medical interventions; to tell them how they can plan ahead for their baby's birth; and, most importantly, to teach them enough so when they say no to unnecessary interventions they can justify their reasoning.

By wisely choosing her provider and support team, a mom can be assured that she'll have ongoing, informed support throughout her birth. This also ensures that mom gets what she wants during labor.

Speaking as a nurse, I strongly support the presence of birth professionals in hospitals and birth centers so moms get help with their labor and birth. Working as a labor and delivery nurse, I'm relieved when a woman comes in with a birth partner. I'm glad to see she has constant help for as long as she's going to be in the hospital. I want every birthing woman to have this kind of support—someone they can trust who will be there for them no matter what.

Because of this desire to inform moms of their need for help, and the need for them to know what risks and side effects medical interventions have, I decided to write this guidebook. I want to help moms find the support they need to make informed decisions for the birth of their baby. I have compiled ideas, knowledge, tips, and insights from all kinds of practitioners—doulas, childbirth educators, massage therapists, acupressurists, midwives, and other birth professionals from across the United States and Canada—and blended them with my own. I want this guidebook to be a portal for pregnant parents that will lead them to well-informed birthing decisions. I hope it will give parents a clear picture of what they want and help make their birth a success by inspiring them to hire a birth professional for labor support and to create a birth plan based on informed decisions. I want to arm pregnant families with enough knowledge and desire to use this information to clearly and confidently tell their practitioner—be it a midwife, physician, naturopath, chiropractor, or others—what kind of birth they truly want—and then stick by it.

How To Use This Book

I put this guidebook together to be just that, a guidebook. I decided not to dwell on any one specific subject (outside of, perhaps, breastfeeding and birth plans, which I feel especially strong about). I'm presenting general information that will introduce to, and hopefully excite you about, all the opportunities that are available to you.

When you first found out you were pregnant, I'm sure you asked yourself many questions: Where do I want my baby born? Who do I want to have there with me? What choices do I have during my labor? How do I go about finding answers? How do I know what's safe for me and my baby during labor?

Chances are that over the months until you give birth you will look at lots of books and talk to lots of people about your pregnancy and pending birth. This guidebook will help by introducing different pregnancy and birthing techniques. Then it will show you how to locate additional help or hire someone for each of the techniques mentioned. Of course, if you are under the care of a physician and receive advice that contradicts advice in this book, challenge your physician, but follow your doctor's advice if the individual characteristics of your problem dictate a different birthing plan.

Writing this book was tremendous fun! I emailed over 1200 birth professionals, doulas, midwives, teachers, RNs, breastfeeding advocates, and many more great women (and yes, some men) who have dedicated their lives to the baby business. The topics I chose were based on two things: what I believe you should read, and what birth attendants consistently brought up. I don't have direct hands-on experience with every suggestion in this guidebook personally, but I have researched them all extensively and recommend them wholeheartedly.

Following is a list of the chapters and a brief description of their contents.

Chapter 1: Home and Hospital Patient Bills of Rights, and Homebirth Bill of Responsibilities

These Bills of Rights are oh, so very important when you enter the hospital in labor. They are lists of rights that you and your baby have. They're common knowledge in the medical field—but not always known by parents. A copy of the Hospital Patient Bill of Rights is nice to bring to the hospital when you're in labor, along with a copy of your birth plan.

I've also included a list of your rights if you birth your baby at home, and there is an important section about your responsibilities as a pregnant parent if you choose to step out of the traditional during your baby's birth.

Chapter 2: Hiring the Help — Physicians, Midwives, and Doulas / Workbooks

This is an important first step after you find out you're pregnant, or if you're planning on getting pregnant. This chapter will give you vital information on how to find, interview, and hire your birthing team.

Your Physician: The first section discusses the hiring of your physician. It gives you ideas of what to ask during the interview, and what to expect from him/her—the person who (after you) is most influential in the outcome of your baby's birth. A workbook is included; after you complete it you'll have a pretty good idea of what's important to you and what type of physician you want to hire.

Your Midwife: The next section outlines how to find and hire a midwife. It explains the various types of midwives that are available and how different each type's role is during your pregnancy and labor. The chapter is filled with questions to ask in the interviewing process, information about what to expect, and material to help you determine who is likely to work best with you. This section also has a workbook that you can fill out and take with you during the interview and decision process.

Your Doula: The last section explains how and why to hire a doula. First, it explains who and what doulas are and how one can assist with your labor, your baby's birth, and even the postpartum period of your pregnancy. This section describes their skills and how to find one through different organizations, and outlines interviewing questions in another workbook.

After reading this chapter you should be able to easily hire the team you want working for you throughout your pregnancy and beyond.

Chapter 3: Medications in Labor / Workbook

This is the most serious chapter in the book—the one that I want you to spend the most time with. As a labor and delivery RN, I feel there isn't nearly enough education offered or information given to pregnant moms about drugs and their side effects. This is a very sensitive subject, so I want everyone who reads this section to do additional research. Lots of it. Many pregnancy and birthing books only glance at the subject of drugs, and providers in the medical industry tend to feel that if they give out too much information it will limit their control of labor. This chapter, however, will give you important information you need to make an informed choice about drugs.

So please read and reread this chapter. Take it to your provider's office and ask them what their views are on drug use. Let them know what you want and when you want it, or simply tell them you don't want anything at all.

I also focus a lot on epidurals—their use is now in epidemic proportions; in the opinion of many people, they are often misused or overused. Narcotics are discussed, and I present the side effects of Pitocin, a drug that's currently very popular in the birthing industry. I try to show you how to make informed choices that will positively affect your labor and your baby's health at birth. The workbook will help you pinpoint exactly what you want and show you how to present that to your provider and hospital staff.

Chapter 4: Herbs in Pregnancy and Childbirth

As we look at complementary methods of birthing we are also looking at optional ways to deal with the discomforts of pregnancy, the management of childbirth, and the care of our bodies and babies in the postpartum phase. This chapter will give you examples, ideas, and a "taste" of how herbs can help you. If the subject interests you, there are books and websites that you can explore listed in the back of this book.

Chapter 5: Complementary Methods of Pregnancy and Labor Management

This chapter will introduce some different options to traditional choices in pregnancy and labor management. It's a fun chapter to explore and covers the arts of HypnoBirthing®, yoga, reflexology, and acupressure in pregnancy and childbirth. These skills are becoming more and more popular and available to pregnant women. The feedback I've received from moms who used these methods has been very positive—they feel their use made their pregnancy and labor easier to manage.

Chapter 6: Vaginal Birth after Cesarean / Workbook

This chapter will help you succeed in a vaginal birth after a cesarean (VBAC). Cesarean operations now account for over 27.6% of births in the United States—far more than anywhere else. And once a mom has a cesarean, she is likely to have a repeat—and likely unnecessary—cesarean unless she is prepared and selective about whom she chooses as her care provider. To be successful with a VBAC it's very important that you be well informed. There are new guidelines being created even as you read this that will make it harder to successfully accomplish a vaginal birth after a cesarean. This chapter will help you create a VBAC birth plan, show you how to choose the right provider and hospital, and give you helpful tips for recovery if you do have a cesarean. The workbook following the chapter will help you put your thoughts together to present to potential providers during the interview process.

Chapter 7: Homebirth / Workbook

I've included homebirth in this book because I feel that to have total control of your labor and your baby's birth this is the route to seriously consider. Homebirths are not for every pregnancy (and I explain why), of course, but if you fit the criteria, then I recommend that you investigate the possibilities and see if it's for you. I introduce statistics comparing hospital births and homebirths, and tell you how to get ready for the homebirth, how to prepare for the unexpected (like having to go to the hospital), and explain what happens during your baby's birth. There's also a wonderful story of a homebirth I attended in Canada. There's a workbook at the end of the chapter that will walk you through your options and show how to create a birth plan that will work for you.

Chapter 8: Waterbirths

Waterbirths are common in Europe and are becoming very popular in the United States as more and more hospital birthing centers offer the option. I've never seen a more gentle and sensual way to birth a baby; the water creates a pleasant and soothing style for labor, and the baby comes out peaceful and content.

Chapter 9: Birth Plans / Workbook

A birth plan is a powerful way to present your desires to your birthing team, and my favorite thing to teach my pregnant couples. It is your written plan presenting what you want to have happen to you and your baby during your stay in the hospital. Creating a birth plan tailored to your needs is usually your doula's greatest strength, so pick her brain on this one. It's everything you desire put into a single contract with your provider. To give it the strength it needs to be effective be sure to have your provider sign it—it then becomes law in the hospital world. There is a great workbook at the end of the chapter. After you've read this chapter you should have a good idea of what you want to have happen during your baby's birth.

Chapter 10: Breastfeeding / Workbook

Ah, the joys of breastfeeding. This chapter is my favorite, and I cover everything that will help you through the beginning of your breastfeeding experience. The chapter is laid out in a question-and-answer format that's ideal for covering so much material. There's a workbook with this one too, and in the back of the book there are several books and websites listed that will help you with any additional questions.

Chapter 11: Birthing Wisdom from Across the Country

This chapter is a blast. These are actual emails that I've received from across the country and Canada concerning every aspect of birthing. You'll find new tips, tricks, and techniques, and want to explore even more.

Chapter 12: Coalition for Improving Maternity Services (CIMS)

This organization provides guidelines for identifying and designing mother-friendly birth sites. Its mission is to improve birth outcomes by promoting a wellness model of maternity care. I love these people; they are making real changes. This chapter will help you find the hospital in your area that follows these guidelines—or comes closest to it. Having this information is a good start to making your hospital and birthing clinics accountable and helping create changes.

Appendix I: Books to Read, and Read Again

This section is divided into sections on Pregnancy and Childbirth, Birthing Choices, Breastfeeding, Vaginal Birth after Cesarean and Cesarean Births, Herbs in Pregnancy and Childbirth, HypnoBirthing and Hypnosis, Yoga and Prenatal Exercises, Reflexology and Acupressure, and Touch and Massage. These authors really know their stuff.

Appendix II: Websites to Surf

This is a listing of websites with information that will be soooo helpful. They will show you where you can find additional information on everything mentioned in this book. Almost all of the websites will link you to others with similar interests. The ones I chose include doula sites, sites constructed by various birth-related organizations, and sites where you can obtain useful information on breastfeeding, HypnoBirthing, yoga, herbs, and childbirth classes. You'll be able to find tons of information about any topic on pregnancy and childbirth—and have fun doing it. Check out their links, and don't forget to bookmark your favorites so you can come back to them. And check our own website at *HeyAnyway.com*.

Appendix III: Contributors

This is a list of many of the birth professionals who offered substantial assistance with this book. You are encouraged to look them up and perhaps consider using their services. I want to thank them so much for the time they spent sharing their wisdom.

So, that's how to use this book and a little bit about what's in it. Exploring your options should be fun. Check out the websites and buy some of the books mentioned in the back. And above all, congratulations on your pregnancy!

Oh my God, you're going to be a mommy!

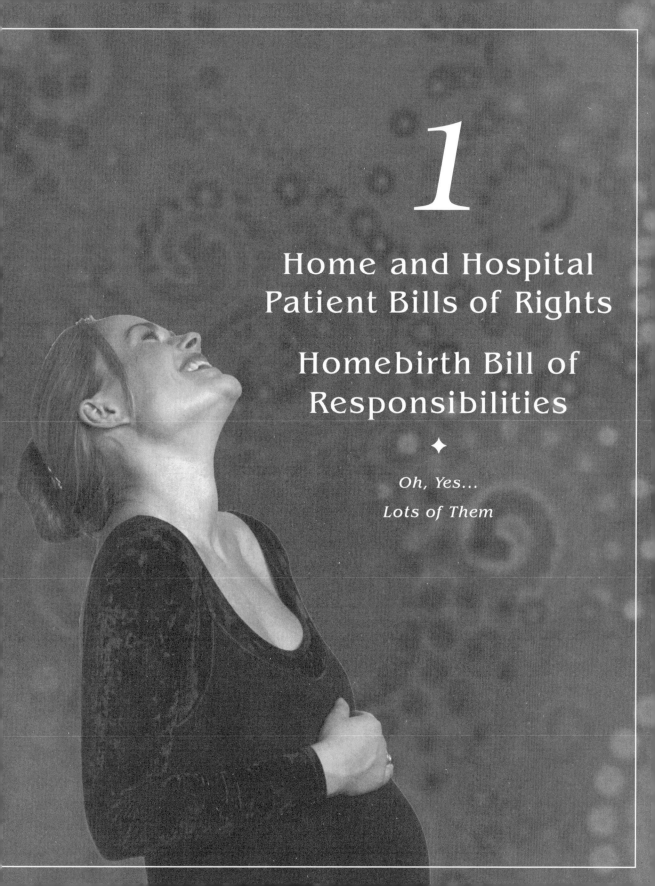

1

Home and Hospital Patient Bills of Rights

Homebirth Bill of Responsibilities

◆

Oh, Yes...
Lots of Them

"A mother always has to think twice—once for herself and once for her child."
　　—Sophia Loren

Women are demanding to be treated differently in hospital birthing rooms than they've been in the past. We're starting to take ownership of our care. We're asking a lot more questions and expecting explanations about procedures. Still, when we enter a medical institution in labor, confused and scared, it's easy to forget we have rights. And with the shortage of nurses and the way we're rushed through each phase of care, these rights aren't always acknowledged. Nevertheless, they must be respected and enforced no matter how much longer it takes the staff to attend to them. No doubt it's easier and quicker for hospital staff to put us through our paces to get procedures done, but as paying patients we have the right to slow things down and know exactly what's going to happen to us and our loved ones.

Following is the Pregnant Patient's Bill of Rights. This is an adaptation of the Patient Bill of Rights compiled by the American Hospital Association It is suited to fit both the pregnant woman and her unborn child.

Pregnant Patient's Bill of Rights

1. You have the right to participate in the development and implementation of your birth plan.

During your pregnancy you can discuss with hospital personnel what you want to have and not have happen to you and your baby throughout your stay, if it's safely possible. You can review your birth plan with the nurse manager and nurses and ask to have it filed in the labor and delivery unit beforehand, and with your medical records at the doctor's office. You can discuss what the hospital doesn't usually do and negotiate ways to make your wishes more possible.

2. You have the right to have the last word regarding the care provided to you and your baby.

If it's hospital policy to remove the baby to the nursery some of the time and you don't want your baby out of your room, you have the final word about saying that your baby stays. During exams, procedures are usually done in the treatment room. If you want your baby treated in your room with you, your request must be considered, or you or your partner have the right to accompany your baby to the treatment room.

3. You have the right to be informed about your health status at any time.

The hospital, nursing, or medical staff can't hold back information about your health or that of your baby. Whenever you ask for results of tests that have been done, no matter how insignificant, the medical staff must find the information and give it to you immediately. They can't expect you to wait for an answer.

4. You have the right to be involved in your treatment, including pain management.

If pain management procedures are not working for you, you have the right to consult with your doctor or pain management technician and help make the decisions that would make your pain manageable. This also applies to any procedure the doctor proposes for the treatment of any ailment you have while hospitalized.

5. You have the right to request that someone of your choice be notified immediately when you're admitted (for example, family members, doula, or your physician).

The hospital can't keep anyone away from you if you have requested that they be present at your birth. If you want to have several members of your family present in the birthing room with you, the hospital must make it possible as long as it's safe. The "immediate family members" rule doesn't apply here. If you want someone present to support you through your birthing process, he or she can't be kept from you. If you signed a waiver to the contrary, of course, this would not be true.

6. You have the right to create a birth plan and expect everyone involved to comply with its directives.

Hospitals are now expecting parents to come in with their own birth plans, and they're bending over backward to comply with their terms. Although some hospitals are still having trouble mustering enthusiasm for some requests, you have the right to present them and work with the nurses to get what you want.

7. You have the right to request or refuse treatment.

If a hospital's policy is to use continuous electronic fetal monitoring during all labors, for example, you have the right to request intermittent monitoring instead if you aren't having problems. If all births include an episiotomy, you can refuse to have one. If stirrups are always used in labor, you can refuse and ask to try without them.

8. You have the right to personal privacy.

This means exactly what it says. If you don't want your name on the report sheet or you don't want to have it known that you're in the hospital, just say so during admission and they must comply.

9. You have the right to choose whom you want in your room and the right to ask visitors to leave before examinations.

When you're admitted to the hospital, let your nurse know whom you want with you throughout your entire labor and your baby's birth and who you'd like to have leave when you're being examined and when you're pushing. The nurse will remember and place a note on your chart so oncoming staff will also know.

10. You have the right to receive care in a safe setting, free from verbal abuse or harassment.

This point needs little explanation. Everyone has a right to feel safe, and if any staff members or any family members make you feel threatened you should immediately report it to the charge nurse or the house supervisor. When you're admitted, most hospitals ask if you feel safe in your environment, and they offer information about shelters and counseling if you're in an abusive relationship.

11. You have the right to the confidentiality of your medical records.

No one other than the medical personnel who are caring for you can have access to your medical records without your permission.

12. You have the right to access information contained in your medical records within a reasonable time frame.

You have the right to get a full copy of your medical record by submitting a signed request at your physician's office or hospital. Although it may take a few days to get copies made, you'll be given them whenever you wish. Your medical records are your property.

13. You have the right to be free from restrictions or forced seclusion used as a means of coercion, discipline, convenience, or retaliation by staff.

No matter how nasty you may become in labor, the staff can't use that behavior against you and treat you differently than they treat someone who is "cooperative" in their eyes.

14. You have the right to be with your baby at all times. If the baby must be examined, the parents have the right to choose who will accompany him or her (e.g., father, doula, midwife).

When hospital personnel take your baby to a treatment room for a test, procedure, or examination and you can't go with them, you have the right to tell the nurse who you want to accompany your baby.

15. You have the right to be treated with respect and dignity.

Yes, yes, and yes!

16. You have the right to file grievances with the hospital.

If you or anyone you're with was treated unfairly, you have the right and are expected to file a grievance. This kind of treatment shouldn't be expected or tolerated.

17. You have the right to file a complaint with your state's Department of Health Services.

If you're not satisfied with the hospital's response to your grievances, you have the right to file a complaint with the Department of Health Services.

Homebirth Bill of Rights

I'm always combing the Internet for websites that support homebirth. One day I came across **"Homebirth Access Sydney,"** where I found the Homebirth Bill of Rights and Homebirth Bill of Responsibilities. The site also includes good information about how to make the homebirth choice, and it bolsters this information with inspiring birth stories. The good folks at **www.homebirthsydney.org** granted me permission to include their bills of rights and responsibilities in my book, for which I am grateful. I'm delighted to pass them along to you. Thank you, Jo Hunter. I've included brief comments of my own with each right. These are similar to the Hospital Bill of Rights and good guidelines for to-be moms.

1. The pregnant woman has the right to choose her place of birth.

You have the right to have your baby in the hospital, at a birthing clinic, in your own home, or the home of someone you feel close to and comfortable with. It's your responsibility, however, to consider some sensible guidelines: you must have ambulance access, you should be no more than thirty minutes away from a hospital, and you must have telephone access for emergencies.

2. The pregnant woman has the right to choose her birth practitioner and to be fully informed about her practitioner's qualifications and experience.

When you're shopping around for a midwife or physician, ask a lot of questions. Seek advice from other women who've had their babies at home. Ask prenatal instructors whom they recommend. At the first appointment with the practitioner of your choice, be very direct and ask about their experience in homebirthing, what qualifications they have, and how many homebirths they have attended. If they seem offended by your questions, they're not the right birth professional for you.

3. The pregnant woman has the right to choose who will be present at her birth and the right to refuse entry or to ask anyone to leave her place of birth.

You can invite whomever you want to be present at your birth, whether you're in the hospital or at home. You can also say no to people you don't feel comfortable with. If a midwife works with a particular doula you don't feel completely comfortable with, ask her to find someone else.

4. The pregnant woman has the right of access to literature and information about birth, particularly homebirth.

This should be a no-brainer. After all, it is the twenty-first century.

5. The pregnant woman has the right to know her practitioner's methods and techniques of birth.

When hiring a birth professional, ask questions. Ask to speak to women whose births they've attended. Find out if they feel comfortable attending a homebirth. Ask what circumstances would cause them to transport you to the hospital. Ask, ask, ask.

6. The pregnant woman has the right to know the approximate costs that will be incurred under her practitioner's care.

Don't be shy about discussing prices before you hire your birth professional. No one likes surprises when it comes to money.

7. The pregnant woman has the right to expect that any information she gives her practitioner will be confidential and not divulged to anyone else without her permission.

In most states it's illegal for your birth professional to discuss your case with anyone if you haven't given permission to beforehand. Ask your caregiver what her policy is on who has access to your records. If she has an open-view mentality you may be able to sign a contract that your record isn't shared without your permission.

8. The pregnant woman has the right to comprehensive prenatal care, including access to standard tests and procedures related to the wellbeing of mother and child.

You have the same rights to all prenatal ("antenatal" in Australia) care, examinations, and tests as a woman who births in a hospital. A birth professional doesn't have the right to treat you any differently because you're not choosing a routine hospital birth.

9. The pregnant woman has the right, prior to the administration of any drug, medication, procedure, or test, to be informed by her practitioner about any direct or indirect effects, risks, or hazards to herself or her unborn or newborn baby.

Before you take medication or accept any prescription, ask what it's for and what side effects and risks are associated with it for both you and your baby. A birth professional is obligated to provide all information you ask for.

10. The pregnant woman has the right to determine for herself whether she will accept the risks inherent in a proposed therapy, test, drug, or procedure.

You have the right to refuse any medication or treatment that a birth professional offers you. Remember, though, that you're responsible for the wellbeing of your baby, and refusing treatment or tests may place your baby in danger.

11. The pregnant woman has the right to choose how she gives birth and to be treated with dignity and consideration at all times so that she feels free to follow her instinctive reactions during birth.

This is especially true if you must be transported to the hospital with a failed homebirth. Medical personnel must treat you no differently than they treat patients that chose to birth their babies in the hospital.

12. The pregnant woman has the right to ancillary medical support when needed.

If you need hospitalization with your baby's birth and ask for support from the community such as hiring an ambulance or seeking admittance into the hospital, you can't be refused assistance. They must provide help whether or not you have insurance or the money in your pocket.

13. The pregnant woman has the right, if transferred to a hospital, to be treated with respect and courtesy, and to be accompanied by her practitioner and the support persons of her choice.

If you're admitted to the hospital for complications, no one can turn away your midwife or other support person that was helping you at home.

14. The pregnant woman has the right, if transferred to a hospital, not to be separated from her baby except for valid medical reasons.

Most, if not all, hospitals are now set up so mother and baby can room together. If the hospital has a nursery and hospital personnel suggest you keep your baby there for whatever reason, you have the right to refuse and keep the baby with you. If your baby needs medical attention and you're too sick to accompany him, you can choose a person to go with him.

15. The pregnant woman has the right to comprehensive postnatal care, including support for the establishment of breastfeeding, assessment and care of her newborn baby, and information about relevant screening tests and registration of birth.

After your baby's birth you're entitled to medical attention and guidance to help you successfully breastfeed. No matter what your income, you can't be refused appropriate immunizations or tests that are offered to newborn babies.

16. The pregnant woman has the right to be informed if there is any known or indicated aspect of her or her baby's care or condition that may cause her or her baby later problems.

All test results must be discussed with you. You're to be informed about any findings that may create complications to your infant in later life.

17. The pregnant woman has the right of access to her and her baby's records and to receive a copy of her and her baby's notes when desired.

You have the right to your and your baby's medical records. A copy of all your medical records for the length of your hospital stay can be obtained from the hospital's medical records office after you submit a signed request. Your midwife can photocopy the records after she has charted all her medical findings about your labor and birth.

18. The pregnant woman has the right, in the event of an unexpected outcome to her pregnancy or birth, to receive all the additional support and services that she needs.

Your hospital community has ongoing support groups for parents of physically challenged babies no matter where or how you had your baby. You have the right to request their services for as long as you and your partner need them. If your area doesn't have a support group, logon to the Internet, use the search engine you prefer (such as www.Google.com), and type in the physical challenge your baby has. The websites found will direct you to organizations that will support you with answers to questions you may have.

19. The pregnant woman has the right to complain and to receive satisfaction from her practitioner.

If you're not satisfied with your care at home or in the hospital, there are channels you can go through to register formal complaints.

Pregnant Women's Homebirth Bill of Responsibilities

Parents who are seeking alternatives in childbirth and are choosing a homebirth must be responsible for themselves, their choices, and their baby. I don't take it lightly when women choose homebirths but don't want to do the necessary work to be successful at it.

The Pregnant Women's Homebirth Bill of Responsibilities from the Homebirth Access Sydney website offers solid guidelines for women who are considering homebirth.

1. The pregnant woman is responsible for learning about the physical, psychological, and emotional process of labor, birth, and postpartum recovery.

Knowledge is power. When you understand what happens to your body during your pregnancy and take time to understand the birthing process, including all the stages of labor and possible complications—both those that occur naturally and those that result from intervention—then you're well on your way to being able to maintain control of your pregnancy. Armed with this knowledge, you'll know what to ask of your practitioner during your prenatal visits, what you can and can't have during labor, and what is safe. For instance, if you're asked to try something that's not on your birth plan—using Pitocin to increase the strength of your contractions, epidurals to ease the pain, or other medications that are not proven to be safe, for example—you would know to refuse as well as understand why.

2. The pregnant woman is responsible for learning about good prenatal birth care so that she may choose the best possible arrangements that suit her individuality and circumstances.

During your pregnancy you should learn about the prenatal care you'll be receiving—why each test is ordered and what the results mean to you and your baby's health. This information enables you to begin planning a birth that will accommodate your needs. If test results show you may have complications during the birth or in the postpartum stages, you may then decide to choose a hospital birth with an obstetrician. This will eliminate having to make in-the-moment decisions during your labor at home.

3. The pregnant woman is responsible for learning about her practitioner's methods, including evaluation of statistics or past cases and talking with other clients.

When you choose a birth partner or physician, you're hiring someone who has preconceived notions about exactly how deliveries should be conducted—in other words, *their* way. For example, some practitioners are "rushers." They don't think twice about breaking your membranes, starting Pitocin, or placing you on a time clock and expecting you to be dilated according to schedule. These birthing professionals recommend or perform many cesareans if women don't meet their expectations.

Midwives and doctors keep records of their births—how many were natural, how many used drugs, and how many resulted in cesarean sections. You have the right to review their statistics; you also have the right to ask for phone numbers of some of their past clients. This will teach you a lot about a practitioner's personality and professional routine.

4. The pregnant woman is responsible for her own emotional and physical wellbeing during pregnancy.

During your pregnancy, you'll want to keep yourself in a state of emotional wellbeing. Your hormones will be active and sometimes make you feel a little crazy with all the different moods you'll go through in a day. This is normal, but it will help if you learn how to relax and are assured that some day you'll feel normal again. Figure out what calms you when you're anxious and what makes you feel better when you're tearful. Teas, certain herbs, relaxation techniques, and lots of reassurance from family and friends can help. Exercise is relaxing and makes you limber and stronger for labor. You can probably find numerous prenatal exercise classes by asking your midwife, checking out the local health food store bulletin board, or exploring the Internet. Staying in tune with your emotions, exercising regularly, and attending prenatal classes will help you prepare for your labor, stay fit, and give you an opportunity to meet other women who are in your same situation.

5. The pregnant woman is responsible for attending her antenatal [prenatal] appointments and informing her practitioner if she is unable to attend.

If you're using a midwife for your prenatal care, you're responsible for keeping your appointments or canceling—if needed—as far ahead of time as you can. Homebirth midwives usually do their prenatal visits in the person's home, and to accomplish this they sometimes must travel long distances. But the bottom line is that it's important to attend all your prenatal visits because they're integral to creating a relationship with your professional birth partner and for making sure everything is fine with you and your baby.

6. The pregnant woman is responsible for her own psychological preparation for homebirth in a society that may be unsupportive or even hostile, especially if the pregnancy results in the death of a baby.

Unfortunately, homebirths aren't well accepted as a natural process in the United States, and the media have a heyday with homebirths that result in complications. Like it or not, choosing to have your baby at home is a political statement. It is also often the best decision for your baby. You therefore must be responsible in all your prenatal care. Though you may have no intention of doing so, you're representing thousands of women and inspiring many more who are undecided about homebirth. Being responsible in your eating habits, exercise, and prenatal visits will virtually ensure that another healthy baby will be born at home naturally and without complications.

7. The pregnant woman is responsible for meeting her practitioner's requirements for preparation for homebirth.

When you choose to have your baby at home you must relinquish some of your care to a homebirth professional. This requires that you be willing to complete the birth professional's requirements to help her make your special day happen safely. You may need to purchase birth supplies, have tests at the medical clinic, and attend birth preparation classes. When clients in my midwifery practice don't show up for prenatal visits, put off laboratory tests that are ordered, or don't collect their supplies, I can't help but anticipate trouble. In those circumstances I usually suggest they birth their first child at the hospital and consider having the next one at home instead. If these parents decide they're truly serious about a homebirth, things usually change. If they don't tend to comply, then it is usually best that they don't birth at home because in their hearts they're not truly ready.

8. The pregnant woman is responsible for informing the practitioner of any relevant physical, emotional, or psychological information that may affect the outcome of her birth.

This information may include use of drugs, medications, herbs, and allopathic, naturopathic, psychological, or alternative therapies as well as the obstetrical, sexual, or psychological history of herself and her relations, friends, or partners that are affecting her attitude about birth and parenting. All or some of this information can determine how labor will proceed, and some will definitely determine how the baby will tolerate the labor and delivery. Information is vital to the birth professional, and it helps tell her if other tests or precautions will be necessary to help her have a safe birth.

9. The pregnant woman is responsible for providing a suitable birth place and healthy environment for her newborn baby.

Choose a place to have your baby that is safe, comfortable, and accessible to emergency vehicles. If you live in the country miles away from a hospital on a dirt road that's inaccessible at the time (in winter, for example), then that is probably not the best place to birth your baby. I know it would be nice to be in your own place, and it will be wonderful after you give birth to retreat to it, but seriously consider finding a friend or family member who lives closer to town who would be willing to make their home your birthing place.

10. The pregnant woman is responsible for making any alternative arrangements for her birth and for being booked into a hospital.

There is always a chance—slim, but a chance—that you'll have to be transported to the hospital for an unforeseen complication or simply because of lack of progress in your labor. Have a backup plan—make arrangements with a doctor of your choice that will come to the hospital and care for you so you won't have to rely on an on-call doctor. Ask your birth practitioner how to pre-register into the hospital, then file a profile and a birth plan with the labor and delivery department. Post near your telephone the numbers of the doctor you choose, the hospital's labor and delivery department, and an ambulance service. These arrangements will help if you're transferred and your labor is still hours away from ending. Remember that once you're in the hospital, the nurse assigned to you is on your side and wants the best outcome for you and your baby. Sometimes when a mother is admitted the midwife wants to stay in total control of the labor and, unfortunately, sometimes this just can't happen. Everyone is a team—the nurse, doctor, and midwife can successfully work together and help you have a healthy baby.

11. The pregnant woman is responsible for making mutually agreed-upon birth plans with her practitioner in advance of labor.

Before your due date you and your partner should sit down with your birth professional and talk about what you want to have happen during your labor and your baby's birth. Talk about pain management, labor breathing and relaxation, birthing styles, and when to transport if you have problems. All of these, discussed ahead of time, will give you a chance to learn what other tips and tricks your midwife may have and acquaint her with what will work best for you.

12. The pregnant woman is responsible for choosing a suitable support person or persons for her birth and for ensuring they are emotionally and psychologically prepared for their role at her birth.

Besides hiring a midwife to attend the birth, some couples also hire a doula or labor coach to help with their laboring process. You may choose family members to be at your labor to care for other children, keep the husband/partner fed, run errands while you're laboring, and just be there to keep things in order. Arrange for these helpers ahead of time and have alternatives in case they're unable to attend when you begin labor.

13. The pregnant woman is responsible for being assertive enough to send away anyone that is not supporting her during her labor.

I have been to many births where for some reason the mother stops laboring or progresses slowly. When I step back and look around the room I sometimes notice that a certain someone is causing the laboring mother to be uncomfortable. Often she doesn't even realize it. When I clear out the room to quiet things down, her labor picks up again and she resumes her work. If someone in the room is annoying you, being too loud, or is making comments that are not helpful, feel free to tell them to leave. You can also tell the midwife or doula and she'll gladly ask them to step out or diplomatically give them a chore that will take them from the room.

14. The pregnant woman is responsible for ensuring that her support people can carry out her preferences if she is unable to express them during labor.

Give all your caregivers your birth plan. Talk to them about what is really important to you and be sure that they'll carry out the plan. For example, if at the last minute you want to have your baby's sibling at your labor, delegate this responsibility to someone. Or if you want to birth your baby in a certain position, be sure that someone is assigned to remind the midwife. Your support caregivers are very important to you, so be sure to communicate all your desires to them.

15. The pregnant woman is responsible for the psychological and emotional preparation of siblings for the birth.

Talk to your other children about your impending birth. Many wonderful books about birthing are available for children. Tell them as much as you can, because at home there's a good chance they'll be present. Don't let the birth process be a surprise to them. If you don't want them at the birth, hire a sitter who can come when you're in labor and take them home with her or him. If you do want them at the birth, hire someone assigned especially to the children. This is no time for the father to be taking care of you while simultaneously trying to watch the kids. The person you assign to be with your other children can help explain all that is going on and, if the kids get bored during labor, can take them away from the premises.

16. The pregnant woman is responsible for the choosing and preparation of individual support people for siblings.

My comments about the preceding point apply here as well. Have someone present whose only responsibility is your children—someone they know and will feel comfortable with.

17. The pregnant woman is responsible for acquiring information about breastfeeding and care of the newborn.

Ask your midwife or physician whom they recommend for breastfeeding instruction. If you live in a larger community, a La Leche League instructor is probably available. Usually the person you hire for prenatal classes can help with breastfeeding advice also. Numerous books about breastfeeding and newborn care are available in bookstores, on the Internet, or in your library. Good old Dr. Spock's classic book, *Baby and Child Care,* and his other books are still around, revised, and as popular and helpful as ever.

18. The pregnant woman is responsible for arranging domestic support for herself and her family during the postnatal period.

Pamper yourself and hire someone to help with the housework. If you can't manage the extra expense post a list of what you need done on the fridge—for instance, laundry, dishes, or a meal cooked. Then, when company comes to see the baby and invariably asks if there's anything they can do, show them the list and ask them to take on a task or two.

19. The pregnant woman is responsible for obtaining information regarding the cost of her care and arranging for payment.

Before you hire your midwife, doula, and special person to baby-sit the siblings, ask about their rates. Then, when applicable, get written contracts so you'll know before you deliver how much everything will cost. You don't need the surprise of a hidden expense because you failed to ask beforehand.

20. The pregnant woman is responsible for evaluating the quality of care she has received and making any dissatisfaction she may feel known to her practitioner.

If your birth went the way you planned, praise your care providers. Letters of thanks and phone calls of appreciation are always welcome. Conversely, if you didn't like something they did during your labor, it's your responsibility to politely tell them what it was. It will make their practice more successful in the future if they know to change something that is annoying or unprofessional.

Summing It Up.

So, that's it. Those are the rights you have as a homebirth candidate and the responsibilities that go along with making this decision. I know this sounds heavy, but birthing at home **is** serious. On the other hand, the rewards soooo much outweigh the reading, preparation, and planning you'll need to do. The joy of laboring at home and having birth professionals come to your place, your family comfortably around you, a garden to walk in, and your own bed to give birth to your son or daughter surrounded with people you love, trust, and know are helping can be amazing. And when it's all over, everyone else leaves and you snuggle in with your baby and your partner and savor the moment.

2

Hiring
the Help

✦

*Physicians
and Midwives
and Doulas...
Oh My!*

"God heals and the doctor takes the fee."
　—Benjamin Franklin

When you conceive you usually have the help of a partner. During pregnancy you usually have the help of a physician or midwife and some friends. But when you give birth you'll want to go hog-wild and hire anyone and everyone for support. That is what this chapter is about—finding the specially trained and awesome people who'll help you through labor, your baby's birth, and then some.

There are three types of birth professionals that I'll introduce here: physician, midwife, and doula. You'll hire at least one of these to be on your team, but I'm hoping you'll have room for all three. Each has unique skills that differ from—yet complement—the others, and the more skills at your disposal the better.

Remember, insurance companies are demanding shorter hospital stays, which is forcing physicians to speed up the birthing process, and during their training physicians are encouraged to initiate medical interventions. The result is an increase of prescribed labor-inducing drugs creating high-risk births. But thank god we live in an age where we're more informed of our options and are getting better advice on how to control our labor. Now, more than ever, it becomes your job to responsibly hire the right professionals that will support your individual wishes. They're out there, and they want to help—all you have to do is invite them along for the ride.

> If after reading *Hey!* you realize that the provider you've already hired isn't working for you, you have the right to fire them. You hired them, you pay their salary, and if you don't like what they are suggesting or what their policies are, then you can find someone else. Firing a provider doesn't mean that you have to confront them. Just find another provider, and have them send for your records. If you want to tell the one you fired what you didn't like about them, send a letter. But keep in mind that no matter how badly you feel for the provider you fired, you did a good job of being a good mommy to your baby.

✦ *PHYSICIANS* ✦

At some time during your pregnancy and labor you'll probably need the services of a physician. You may want him or her to attend your birth or, if you're having a homebirth with a midwife, you'll need a backup physician in case complications upset your plans. In either case it's in your best interests to do some research and conduct some interviews to determine which physician is the best match for you.

In 300 B.C., a gynecologist was put on trial for cross-dressing and practicing medicine:

Women were not allowed to attend medical school, so Agnodice got around this by impersonating a male student. She continued this practice afterwards until one of her patients did not want a "man" to examine her. So Agnodice disrobed and revealed her real gender. She was put on trial for practicing medicine while female. The townspeople mobbed the trial and pleaded for her life.

She was pardoned.

There are all sorts of doctors that attend births. Some are in family practice and can take care of you, your baby, and the whole family; some specialize in newborns or toddles only. They come in all shapes and sizes, and they practice just as differently.

Obstetricians/gynecologists (OB/GYNs) can help you manage your pregnancy and labor. A pediatrician will care for your baby after you have her. Some doctors have large practices with lots of other physicians, and a different one may be on duty every night of the week. (When you go into labor you may not know who's on call, so you need to meet them all.) Some physicians have a smaller practice and even work with a midwife or doula that will be available during your labor. Some work exclusively from the hospital, and others have a birthing clinic or a small birthing suite in their office. With all these options to consider, you'll need to start looking for a physician early in your pregnancy. Whether you're planning a homebirth, a hospital birth, or to have your baby in a birth clinic, hire a doctor who will work in your best interests.

First, sit down with your partner, doula, midwife, and/or parents and discuss what options you have and what kind of physician would work best for you and your baby. Talk to friends with babies as well as the labor and delivery nurses at your hospital. Talk to certified lactation consultants—they know which physicians support breastfeeding. Talk to local prenatal instructors and midwives; even if you aren't planning a homebirth they know who is open minded about natural childbirth. If you want an epidural, find out which anesthesiologist is best. Find a doctor who is willing to let you dilate to at least 5–7 centimeters before considering an epidural.

What To Consider

Is the physician:

✦ available throughout your entire pregnancy?

✦ open minded and flexible? Does he want his own way and has he been practicing so long that he is unwilling to change, or is he willing to try things that are new and somewhat out of the norm?

✦ supportive of midwives? Does this physician flip out when you mention that you want a midwife at your birth?

✦ knowledgeable about doula services? Does he know what a doula is? Does he work with doulas or know ones you can contact for coaching during your labor?

✦ willing to listen to your ideas? Are you given time to say what you want? Does he seem to be truly listening to what you're saying or is he rushing you out of the office?

✦ in a position to offer classes? Does his staff offer prenatal or breastfeeding classes before you start labor?

✦ supportive of breastfeeding? This is a must, because if he supports your choice, he'll have all the access you need to be a successful breastfeeder.

✦ working with a friendly and supportive staff? You may find the perfect physician who is friendly and supportive, but he may have the staff from hell that are disrespectful, short tempered, and unhelpful. This would kill your relationship with the physician.

✦ in practice with partners who believe the way he does? When you hire a physician in a large practice, you're also hiring his partners. If his partners don't think the same way he does, are they willing to bend their beliefs to accommodate you?

◆ willing to give you the time you need? Do office appointments last longer then fifteen minutes, or do you feel you're wasting his time when you're with him? Does he act as if you're important to him?

◆ willing to review your birth plan with you and sign it so it becomes his orders when you enter the hospital?

When you've done your homework and located several possibilities, narrow your search down to a couple of physicians and make appointments with them. Tell the receptionist that you're considering hiring the physician and want to set up an interview. This is usually a free visit, and you should be given a good thirty minutes to ask questions.

Remember, the physician is your employee. You're his boss, and he's working for you, so treat the situation accordingly. There's no need to be aggressive or disrespectful; however you must state what you expect from a physician and that you won't compromise matters that are important to you.

First Impressions

What does the physician's office look like? Is it arranged with the patient in mind? Are there birthing magazines, brochures, and fliers about local childbirth classes, and breastfeeding support pamphlets in the waiting room? Are the chairs comfortable and the room clean and well lit? These considerations may sound trivial, but if the doctor wants to make a good first impression, then he's probably interested in keeping you as a client too.

How long are you kept waiting for your interview? If you're kept waiting by a physician who'll later be billing you a significant amount, how will he treat you when you're his client?

When you meet the doctor face to face, does he stand up when you enter the room? Does he shake your hand? Does he look you in the eye and call you by name? If you're with your husband/partner, does he know their name too? If so, it indicates that he did his research before you arrived—a good sign. Does he treat you like a couple, addressing both of you with his answers and comments?

If your partner is not with you, bring someone else to help you remember questions and the doctor's answers. Someone with medical or birth experience would have a particularly helpful perspective.

What To Ask

General Questions: After you've introduced yourselves and exchanged pleasantries, it's time to relax and start asking questions.

What is your fee?
Before you develop a relationship with this physician, ask about his fees. What exactly do the charges cover, and how does he like to be paid? Does his practice accommodate your insurance company? Does he want your bill to be paid in full before you give birth? Does he accept payments?

What is your experience?
Has he always worked in a hospital, or has he attended home and clinic births as well? This could really influence the outcome of your birth. If you want a very natural birth and he has only worked in hospitals and has only experienced births that are intervened, that may be what he calls natural.

What is your philosophy about childbirth?
It's important to know what his priorities are for making your birth successful and what he considers a successful birth.

According to recent American Medical Association figures, the average patient waits 19 minutes for a scheduled appointment with a doctor and he will interrupt you an average of every eleven seconds.

Do you have partners? May I meet them too?
Most practices have partners, and they usually share the same philosophy. But it's a good idea to meet with them, show them your birth plan, and make sure they'll try to abide by it too.

Does your staff teach prenatal classes or breastfeeding classes?
Do you employ midwives or doulas?
It's great when a physician takes the time and interest to hire midwives and doulas and offers prenatal classes or classes on breastfeeding. It's even better when he insists that you take the classes.

What tests and initial prenatal care do you offer?
Does he insist on an ultrasound with each visit? Frequent ultrasounds are becoming the norm with some obstetricians. However research is showing that more than a couple of ultrasounds throughout pregnancy are unsafe.[1] What lab work does he order, and what is he looking for?

What are your parameters for weight gain?
Normal weight gain for the average-size woman is 25–35 pounds. For overweight women it's 15–25 pounds and if under-weight, 28–40.

What do you consider a full-term pregnancy?
Term is considered 38–42 weeks. If your physician considers inducing only a couple of days over 40 weeks, tell him "no way" unless it is medically warranted.

How do you induce labor?
Does he use internal vaginal inserts first or does he want to start right away with the big guns like Pitocin?

If I am considering a homebirth, how early and late can I have my baby at home?
Does he base his decision on statistics or by how well you and the baby are doing?

Who will provide prenatal care?
Does he see you on each visit, or does he have an assistant who does all the prenatal care? How often will you be seen?

During prenatal care, what conditions would classify me as high risk?
When your physician starts talking to you about being high risk, have him take the time to show you statistics and facts that back up his thinking. Being placed in a high risk category during your pregnancy can create the need for additional tests, ultrasounds, and precautions that will follow you into the hospital and create an array of situations that may go against your desires.

What percentage of labor inductions have you done in the last year and why? What percentage of epidurals? Cesareans?
This is very important to know. It will indicate his mindset, patience, and ability to birth a woman naturally.

How long after my membranes rupture am I expected to start labor?
It's policy to have your baby within 24 hours after your membranes rupture. But this isn't etched in stone, so don't let it be a deciding factor for induction. If your physician insists on induction, have him show you statistics that prove that infection will start by 24 hours after rupture.

What methods would you use, besides Pitocin, to stimulate labor?
You need to know if your physician will consider other choices for induction besides Pitocin, such as reflexology, herbs, massage oils, or acupressure.

Do you use routine IVs or saline locks?
Starting an IV or saline lock only makes introducing other drugs easier to justify if the physician doesn't feel your labor is going textbook perfect. Delay this as long as you can.

How about intermittent fetal monitoring?
You don't need to be on a monitor all the time. Ask to be only intermittently monitored during your labor so you can get up, walk around, leave the room, or take a shower or a nice long bath.

Will you allow me to eat when I want?
Food offers nourishment. You have to eat and drink for strength. If you puke, you puke, but you still need the calories for energy to help you through labor.

What do you recommend for pain management?
My thought on this is: be wary of any physician who automatically dishes out drugs for pain management. It would be ideal if he recommends breathing and relaxation, position changes, the shower/tub, or other methods before resorting to drugs.

Do you discourage the use of epidurals and Pitocin to speed things up?
It would be a good thing to find a physician that won't rush you through labor. I know some of these physicians, and I admire them.

Can anyone of my choosing be with me during my labor
and my baby's birth?
This is pretty much the case now, but it's still a good question to ask. Some physicians and hospitals will only allow a few people in your room during labor.

Do you allow labor in a tub and birthing in positions other than on my
back with my feet in stirrups?
Many physicians will say you can have your baby in any position you want, but when pushing time comes they usually want you on your back with your bottom scooted to the edge of the bed while they sit on a stool waiting to catch. If you agreed on other positions, make sure your partner holds him to it.

Will my baby, if not in distress, be placed on my abdomen immediately after the birth? May I nurse within an hour after he's born? Can baby's examinations and procedures (e.g., eye ointments, vitamin K shots) be done while I'm present? Does the hospital you deliver at follow mother-friendly protocols? How many of your patients breastfeed?

Take these questions to your physician, and talk to the nurse manager of the hospital where you're going to labor. They'll let you know what their policy is (each hospital is different).

Will you provide me with the phone numbers of other women whose births you have attended?

Ask; this shouldn't be a problem.

Homebirth-Related Questions

If you are planning a homebirth, you should still engage the services of a physician in case you have to be admitted to the hospital for an unforeseen complication. You'll receive most of your prenatal care from your midwife and visit the backup physician once for an introduction and interview. It's to your benefit to choose a physician who supports homebirth so that your transition into the hospital, if needed, goes smoothly and you're treated with dignity and respect. An on-call physician in the hospital may not support your wishes. You may also encounter problems with the nursing staff because many aren't sympathetic toward women who transport from a homebirth. This is unfortunate, because they have an opportunity to learn a lot from the midwives who bring the mothers in; and the midwives could learn from the nursing staff too.

Your midwife could probably recommend a backup physician or two who she's worked with in the past. Make an appointment with one of them, give him a copy of your medical record, and let him know what your desires are if you should end up in the hospital.

Here are some questions you may want to ask your backup physician.

✦ Do you support my desire to birth my baby at home? What are your concerns about my choice? What can I do to make my homebirth plans more acceptable to you?

✦ Do you want me to call you when I start labor?

✦ Would you like to have more than one visit with me before I go into labor?

✦ Do you want all my lab work faxed to your office for your records, or should I simply contact you if there are any abnormalities?

✦ If you haven't already done so, would you like to meet my midwife?

✦ If I am having concerns during my labor, would you be willing to come to my home instead of expecting me to go to the hospital?

✦ Would you be willing, if it could be done safely, to continue keeping my birth as natural as possible in the hospital and not routinely order lab tests, IVs, medications, and other interventions?

✦ If the birth went well and there are no complications, would you consider a discharge at six hours?

This should give you an idea on how to find a physician you can work with. You may not find a physician that fits your criteria perfectly, but the information you've gathered will make it much easier to make a good choice. Don't forget, you're the boss, you know what you want, and there's no need to compromise your wishes. Stay informed about your lab results and trust that everything will go according to plan.

Hiring A Physician

Hiring a physician is hard—not only are you hiring someone for yourself and what may ail you during your pregnancy, but you're hiring someone to take care of your baby while you're pregnant. While making up your mind you and your partner need to be thinking of the same plan. Go over these questions together, get straight what exactly you're looking for in a physician, and then use the information when you interview.

Below is a place to put some phone numbers of physicians that you're considering.

Name _____

Telephone _____

Office Address _____

_____

Hospital _____

Name _____

Telephone _____

Office Address _____

_____

Hospital _____

Name _____

Telephone _____

Office Address _____

_____

Hospital _____

Name _____

Telephone _____

Office Address _____

_____

Hospital _____

Name _____

Telephone _____

Office Address _____

_____

Hospital _____

Name _____

Telephone _____

Office Address _____

_____

Hospital _____

What You're Looking For in a Physician

Now to start exploring what will work for you. Here's a quick recap of what we covered in the physicians section of the Hiring the Help chapter.

		Yes	No
1.	Do you want to hire a:		

❏ Family practice physician   ❏ Obstetrician

Note: It is important to know that these are two different types of practice. They both help birth babies, but the obstetrician is a surgeon—with a different mentality when labor isn't textbook perfect.

		Yes	No
2.	I want a physician who has a large practice.	❏	❏
3.	I care if my physician is male or female.	❏	❏
4.	It is important that my physician has the support of birth professionals, including midwives and doulas.	❏	❏
5.	I need the support of a breastfeeding advocate available through his office.	❏	❏
6.	If he has partners I want to meet them.	❏	❏
7.	I want my physician to read, agree to, and sign my birth plan.	❏	❏

8. I want my physician to be
    (check all that are important to you):

❏ Young

❏ Older (experienced)

❏ Professional all the time

❏ Just hospital oriented (not doing home or clinic births)

❏ In control

❏ Open to my ideas

❏ Willing to change his ideas on some things

❏ Available by phone

Physician's Office

	Yes	No
9. Is the office close to my home?	❏	❏
10. Is the office close to the hospital?	❏	❏

11. What do I think of the staff when I visit or call?

_____

_____

12. When I call I want to have available by phone
(if I have questions):

❏ Nurses   ❏ Doulas
❏ Breastfeeding advocates   ❏ Just a receptionist

	Yes	No
13. I don't need prenatal classes offered by the physician's office; I will seek my own.	❏	❏
14. I hate waiting in the doctor's office for my appointment.	❏	❏
15. It is important in non-emergent cases to have available next-day appointments.	❏	❏
16. I prefer that there be a laboratory in the office to do routine lab work.	❏	❏
17. I prefer that the office have an ultrasound available.	❏	❏

Questions For The Interview

		Yes	No
1.	I want to know all about your experience.	❏	❏
2.	I care if you have experience in home or clinic births.	❏	❏
3.	I want to know your philosophy about childbirth.	❏	❏
4.	I don't have insurance. I need to make arrangements with your office for payment.	❏	❏
5.	I don't want routine lab work done unless necessary.	❏	❏
6.	I don't want an ultrasound at every visit. I understand this isn't necessary and may be dangerous to the baby.	❏	❏
7.	I don't want induction for elective reasons even if I'm tired of being pregnant.	❏	❏

8. If I am told I must be induced I want to first try:

   ❏ Nipple stimulation   ❏ Acupressure

   ❏ Reflexology   ❏ Herbs

9. I want "premature" considered to be before _____ weeks and "postdates" considered to be after _____ weeks.

10. How many inductions have you done, and why?

   _____

11. How many ruptured membranes, and why?

   _____

12. How many cesareans, and why?

   _____

13. How many epidurals, and why?

   _____

Yes   No

14. Do you encourage epidurals? Why or why not?

_____

15. How many natural (no medications at all) births
     have you done?

_____

16. What other positions besides lithotomy do you
     encourage during the pushing stages?

_____

17. Are you willing to let me push:

On my side   ❏   ❏

Squatting   ❏   ❏

Hands and knees   ❏   ❏

Standing   ❏   ❏

18. I would like to have some phone numbers
     of other women you have attended:

Name/Phone _____

Name/Phone _____

Name/Phone _____

Home Birth Questions

Yes   No

19. Do you support and encourage homebirths?   ❏   ❏

20. With a midwife present, I want you standing by.
     You will be called if there's a need for your presence. ❏   ❏

21. Do you keep a record of all the lab work
     my midwife orders?   ❏   ❏

		Yes	No
22.	Do I have a prenatal visit with you before I begin labor?	❏	❏
23.	Do you personally attend all homebirths that are admitted to the hospital, or rely on your colleagues if you aren't on call?	❏	❏
24.	Would you be willing to come to the home if there are concerns instead of automatically transferring me to the hospital?	❏	❏
25.	If I do go to the hospital, would you try to keep the birth as natural as possible and not rely on routine procedures to control the labor or birth?	❏	❏
26.	Would you consider early discharge after 6 hours if all is well with me and my baby?	❏	❏
27.	Would you be willing to conduct my postpartum checks at my house instead of your office if I need to have a repeat visit?	❏	❏

Other questions I may want to ask:

_____

_____

_____

_____

_____

_____

_____

_____

_____

WORKSHEET ❖ PHYSICIANS

✦ *MIDWIVES* ✦

If you're healthy, receiving good prenatal care, and your pregnancy has been uneventful and is expected to remain so, you may decide to birth your baby at home. Because few physicians agree to attend homebirths, it's likely a midwife will be with you at your birth instead. This chapter will tell you about your choices and suggest questions you can ask to help you find the right midwife for you.

The midwifery profession is made up of various kinds of practices, various levels of experience, and distinct birthing skills. A *Direct-Entry Midwife* (DEM) is a healthcare practitioner educated in the discipline of midwifery through self-directed study, apprenticeship, a midwifery school, a university-based program distinct from the discipline of nursing, or combinations of these. In most situations, because of where they live and the limited availability of schools, DEMs are educated by other direct entry midwives, who then pass along their skills to future midwives. Their training is largely hands-on, with plenty of reading, workshop and conference attendance, participation in discussion groups, and consultations with midwives and doctors.

In 1915, the Association for the Study and Prevention of Infant Mortality published a paper in which Dr. Joseph DeLee described childbirth as a pathologic process. He believed that childbirth was not a normal function and that midwives had no place in childbirth.

An interested woman usually starts her training by observing births attended by a skilled midwife. Her goal is to absorb as much information as she can. When she feels ready, she moves on to the next level—perhaps labor coaching, taking the mother's blood pressure and tracking her heart rate, then learning breathing and relaxation techniques and how to manage fetal heart tones. All the while she's reading and watching birth videos, attending meetings with mentors and homebirth physicians, and taking part in discussion groups. Eventually she'll be "catching" babies, performing baby assessments, and medically managing the mother and baby after she gives birth. This course of education and experience qualifies her to be a direct entry midwife.

An aspiring midwife may decide to attend a direct entry midwifery school and become a *Licensed Direct-Entry Midwife* (LDM). For example, the School of Midwifery in Eugene, Oregon, offers an extensive curriculum that includes study modules in anatomy and physiology, cell biology, embryology and fetal development, nutrition, homeopathy, and prenatal care that includes pelvic exams, labs, and antenatal diagnosis. The capable LDMs who have implemented and been trainers in this program have made homebirths safer and have provided a wonderful service to their community and all of Oregon.

Many women choose the *Certified Nurse Midwife* (CNM) route, which requires that they first complete nursing school to become a registered nurse, and then an accredited program of study and clinical experience in obstetrical care to receive a certified nurse midwifery license. Some states accept candidates into their program who have an associate degree, while others require a bachelor's degree or even a Master's degree. These midwives can practice in hospital and birthing clinics, public health clinics, community health centers, and private practice. Their skills allow them to offer gynecological services such as Pap smears and breast examinations, advise women about reproductive health and personal care, and monitor the health of the mother and fetus during pregnancy. They also provide complete prenatal care, including abdominal and pelvic examinations and evaluations. They seldom attend homebirths because the cost of malpractice insurance is prohibitively high.

> A CNM's license allows her to provide:
> + Preconception care
> + Prenatal care
> + Labor and birth management
> + Postpartum care
> + Routine annual exams (Pap smears and breast exams)
> + Family planning help
> + Treatment for vaginal infections and other gynecological problems
> + Sexuality and contraceptives counseling for adolescents
> + Hormone replacement therapy

A direct entry midwife who is self-taught through reading and apprenticing with an LDM can practice homebirths and possibly attend births at small rural birthing clinics, but can't practice in hospitals or large birth clinics. CNMs who have more clinical study under their belts and six to nine years of college-level nursing and midwifery training can only work in hospitals and birth clinics. In most instances their license is threatened if they attend homebirths. The irony here is amazing: in each case the midwives have developed their skills to an art, and yet they are restricted from using these skills where their particular kind of education and training are especially needed.[1]

In some states it's legal for anyone to call themselves a midwife, whether they have attended ten or a thousand homebirths. These unqualified midwives can really mess up birth-outcome statistics, causing many to claim that all babies should be born in a hospital and homebirth should be illegal.

Speaking as a midwife, I'm a strong supporter of homebirth, especially after my work in labor and delivery at a hospital. If a woman is healthy, well informed about pregnancy and childbirth, determined to avoid medical interventions, and has a good support system and a well-trained midwife on her side, there's no reason she shouldn't birth her baby at home. And here's a good reason why she should: A study conducted by Dr. Lewis Mehl compared matched populations of 2,092 homebirths and 2,092 hospital births. Midwives and family doctors attended the homebirths, and OB/GYNs and family doctors attended the hospital births. Within the hospital group, the fetal distress rate was six times higher, the incidence of maternal hemorrhage was three times higher, limp and unresponsive newborns arrived three times more often, and thirty permanent birth injuries were caused by doctors. In another study, Dr. Mehl compared matched groups of 1,046 homebirths with 1,046 hospital births. There was no difference in infant mortality, but in the hospital there was greater incidence of fetal distress, lacerations to the mother, neonatal infections, forceps birth and cesarean sections, and nine times as many episiotomies.[2]

> In 2001 there were 4,025,933 babies born in the United States:
>
> ✦ 0.07% were caught by CNMs at residences (3,004 babies)
>
> ✦ 0.23% were caught by other midwives at residences (9,651 babies)
>
> ✦ 91.3% were birthed by doctors in hospitals (98.7% in 1975)
>
> ✦ Midwives caught 8% of the babies born in homes, hospitals, etc. (1% in 1975)
>
> *Information gathered from the National Center for Health Statistics*

So are you perfectly safe having your baby at home? Certified childbirth educator and author Carl Jones, in his book *Alternative Birth*, says that, just as there are in all of life, there are always risks during childbirth, so women need to be checked for health problems that "could be dangerous during labor and delivery." He affirms that, "For some women, in rare circumstances, obstetric care is essential," but he also affirms that most mothers will see "better, healthier results" when they "choose to birth at home." So, if you're healthy, consider birthing at home—the risks for both you and your baby are almost always lower.

Finding the Perfect Midwife for You

Because midwives have varying levels of expertise and unique styles, it is important to choose a midwife that you feel is confident and compatible. The following questions may help you select a midwife who is well suited to you and your family:

How did you become a midwife?

Some midwives are self-taught and often start out as prenatal instructors. By reading, attending workshops and conferences, attending births with other midwives, and studying numerous hours, they slowly progress to competent baby-catchers. Midwives who work in hospitals and birthing clinics are first registered nurses who continue their education in a school of midwifery and receive their certified nurse midwifery license. They usually work exclusively in hospitals or clinics, and their license doesn't apply to homebirth situations.

What training have you had?

Some women have attended one or two births and are calling themselves midwives. Get references, talk to women whose births she's attended, and ask your area hospital about her transport rate and if they like working with her. Your and your baby's health and safety depend on this woman, so be sure you know how much she knows.

Are you certified or licensed with any organizations?

Who has certified her education? Is she licensed in your state? Is she a supportive member of a homebirth organization?

Do you belong to any midwifery organizations, attend conferences and workshops, and subscribe to professional journals?

Don't be afraid to ask what conferences and workshops she's attended recently. Ask her what material she's subscribing to that keeps her updated about current tests, studies, and maternal management.

What is your basic philosophy of childbirth?

Ask what is important to her about the birthing process. What are her priorities regarding childbirth?

How many births have you attended as the primary midwife?

Some birth attendants play only a secondary role at births and yet say they have attended a lot of births. In reality they may have been in charge of only a few and have caught only half of those. A primary midwife is responsible for labor management, the birth, conducting the well-baby check, and recognizing complications and notifying the doctor if needed.

Do you handle higher-risk situations, such as twins or breeches?

Many things can go wrong with a twins or breech homebirth, so such situations are usually best managed in a hospital setting. But if the midwife you're interviewing has knowledge and experience in these areas, it is definitely a plus to consider.

What is the fee for your services, how must it be paid, and what does it include?

Get this information right up front. Talk about the fee, all the costs and expenses, and any additional charges she may ask for her services.

What kinds of services are included in your prenatal care?

Does she have access to and privileges at a local laboratory so she can track your blood and urine levels, which will help her detect potential problems during your pregnancy? Some midwives work with a doctor who can process lab work for them. Is she capable of detecting problems early in the pregnancy? Does she offer nutrition information, exercise recommendations, in-home care, or recommendations for parent education via books, videos, or classes?

Do you work with another midwife or assistant at births?

A homebirth requires two sets of hands: one pair for the mother during the baby's birth and the other pair for the baby. A birth attended by a solo midwife is not always safe. For example, if the baby is in trouble and the mother starts to bleed, one person can't handle both situations.

What do you do if two births are about to happen at the same time?

Find out who her backup will be if she has another birth at the same time as yours.

How do I reach you? Do you have a pager that enables 24-hour access?

Find out how to get in touch with your midwife around the clock, either by calling her cell phone, home phone, pager, or backup physician.

How do you handle problems or complications that might develop during labor?

Who is her backup? Does she have access to the local hospital? Is the hospital staff hostile to transports who were attempting a homebirth? Does she have a doctor who supports her and backs her up during emergencies? Can she easily access someone to consult with or, better yet, does someone accompany her to births?

What standard and emergency equipment do you carry? What herbs or medicine do you use? Which ones do you not carry and why?

Some things are important to have handy at a birth: oxygen for the mom or baby if needed, herbal or medicinal intervention for excessive bleeding, vitamin K and erythromycin for the baby's eyes, etc. Find out what your state allows as well as forbids midwives to use. You can obtain this information at *www.cfmidwifery.org/states*.

Are you affiliated with a physician who can answer unusual questions either during the pregnancy or in an emergency?

Don't choose a midwife who doesn't have a backup doctor. When a second opinion is needed, she may not have time to look it up in a medical text. Access to a doctor who'll advise her is a must. In addition, an on-call doctor who is a stranger and who does not support homebirth may be assigned to care for you after a transport—not a pleasant experience.

What is your policy for transporting to a hospital?

If you must be transported, how would she handle it? What medical facilities does she support if complications arise? Does she use a different one during the day, such as a birthing clinic, and the hospital at night? Does she have a doctor who'll meet you "at the door" of the hospital? Does she have good rapport with the hospital? What would make her want to transport you? What does she say she can handle at home? Is she a safe midwife who transports before an emergency develops? Is she respected in the community?

What kind of postpartum care do you provide (frequency of baby checkups or assistance with nursing, for example)?

A midwife should follow up with you after you give birth. She should come to your home at least twice a day for the first couple of days to make sure you're doing well. She should assess your blood flow and establish that your uterus is firm by pressing on your lower abdomen and feeling for it, and help you establish breastfeeding. Some midwives help cook the first meals and help the baby's siblings accept the new family situation. You may want to consider hiring a postpartum doula to help with your care after you have your baby.

Conclusion

Consider everything that is most important to you as you look for a midwife to care for you and your baby. Tell her what you want to have happen during the birth and tell her your fears. Let her know that you're reading and tell her how you're preparing for this special day. Assure her that you love learning as much as you can about your pregnancy and birth, and ask for suggestions about what to read. Find out if she has a lending library.

After interviewing several midwives, set aside open-ended time with your partner to discuss what you liked and didn't like about each one, how each midwife answered your questions, and how you feel in your hearts. Rest assured that you'll find the right midwife for you. Then, allow her to be your guide through the birthing process.

Above all else, having a midwife is like having a new best friend who knows exactly what you're going through. During your prenatal care and the planning for your baby's birth the two of you will develop a friendship that could last a long time. Your midwife will be your teacher, confidant, coach, and advisor. She'll help bring your baby into the world with a gentle touch and a soothing voice. It's a special, intimate relationship that you'll never forget.

Sandra Botting, the midwife I choose to attend my daughters' births, became my mentor and taught me the art of midwifery. She was my guide and guru while I was pregnant and became my best friend, teacher, and partner when I started catching babies myself. We had an almost magical time together catching babies and teaching prenatal classes for years. She'll always have a special place in my heart.

I have met lots of midwives over the last 27 years; there is a special caring and loving feeling you get when you meet one. I hope you can find that in the midwife you hire for your very, very special day.

And when your birth is only a memory and your baby is in your arms, email me all about it. I really want to hear your story.

Hiring a Midwife

This is a little harder then hiring a physician—in most areas there aren't many midwives to choose from and they don't always advertise in the phone book. It will take some research on your part to find one. Check in the back of this book under websites; there are listings to help you find a midwife in your area. Or try the local health food stores, call prenatal instructors, contact local hospitals, and just ask around. When you do locate a few, complete the worksheet below. Good luck.

Start with names, phone numbers, and addresses:

Name _____

Telephone _____

Address _____

_____

Name _____

Telephone _____

Address _____

_____

Name _____

Telephone _____

Address _____

_____

Name _____

Telephone _____

Address _____

_____

Name _____

Telephone _____

Address _____

_____

Name _____

Telephone _____

Address _____

_____

The Interview

Okay, you've collected some phone numbers and made appointments with some of the midwives. Now you and your partner need to sit down and discuss what is important to you. Here are some questions to consider asking the prospective midwives:

	Yes	No

1. How did you become a midwife?

_____

Are you a Certified Nurse Midwife (CNM)? ❑ ❑

Where did you get your training?

_____

Do you also work in a clinic? ❑ ❑

Are you a Direct-Entry Midwife (DEM)? ❑ ❑

Who trained you and how?

_____

How much experience do you have?

_____

How many births have you attended?

_____

How many births were you in charge of?

_____

Are you a Licensed Direct-Entry Midwife (LDM)? ❑ ❑

Where did you go to school?

_____

Is the program recognized in this state? ❑ ❑

How long have you been practicing?

_____

	Yes	No

2.   What is your philosophy of childbirth?

_____

3.   Do you handle high-risk births?   ❑ ❑

How many have you done?

_____

4.   What is your fee?

_____

What does it include?

_____

How do you like to be paid?

_____

5.   Do you do all prenatal care?   ❑ ❑

6.   Do you do labs and ultrasounds if needed?   ❑ ❑

If not, where do I go to have lab work done?

_____

7.   Do you work alone?   ❑ ❑

If not, who do you work with?

_____

8.   Who is your backup physician?

_____

Does he come to the home?   ❑ ❑

9.   Who will cover the birth if you are at another?

_____

What does she charge?

_____

	Yes	No

10. How do I reach you?

   _____

    Do you have a pager or cell phone?   ❑ ❑

    Are you available 24 hours a day?   ❑ ❑

11. Does the local hospital openly accept your homebirthing patients that have to be brought in?   ❑ ❑

12. What emergency equipment do you bring with you?

   _____

13. Do you have a physician you can ask questions of?   ❑ ❑

    If so, who is the physician?

   _____

14. How would you transport me to the hospital if it became necessary?

   _____

    Under what circumstances would you transport me?

   _____

15. Do you offer postpartum care?   ❑ ❑

    If so, what do you offer?

   _____

16. Names and phone numbers of some women you've attended.

    Name _____ Telephone _____

    Name _____ Telephone _____

    Name _____ Telephone _____

    Name _____ Telephone _____

    Name _____ Telephone _____

Typical Things My Midwife Needs To Know

		Yes	No
1.	I don't need prenatal classes taught by my midwife. I have my own prenatal instructor.	❏	❏
2.	I want my lab work done by her backup physician.	❏	❏
3.	I don't need prenatal care from my midwife; I just want her to attend my birth.	❏	❏
4.	I don't want her to bring a trainee to my birth.	❏	❏
5.	I don't want her to bring more than one other person to my birth.	❏	❏
6.	I don't need her during my early labor. I'll have my husband and/or friends coach me.	❏	❏
7.	I would like several prenatal visits at my home to help me set up and arrange things.	❏	❏
8.	I want the room very warm with very low lights for the sake of the baby.	❏	❏

9. I want only these people with me during the actual birth:

_____

_____

_____

		Yes	No
10.	I want to try different positions while pushing.	❏	❏
11.	If, at all possible, I would like my partner to help catch the baby.	❏	❏
12.	I would like _____ to cut the baby's cord.		
13.	I would like to breastfeed right away.	❏	❏
14.	I want siblings at the actual birth.	❏	❏

	Yes	No

15. I want the placenta to come at its own time—
not forced or tugged out.   ❏   ❏

16. I don't need help with breastfeeding after the baby is
born. I have someone who will help me with this already.   ❏   ❏

17. I want postpartum care after the baby is born.   ❏   ❏

18. I would like _____ visits after my baby is born and
would like you to come by for _____ days to check
on my progress.

19. I would like phone numbers of people who can help me with
breastfeeding and postpartum care.

Name _____ Telephone _____

Name _____ Telephone _____

Name _____ Telephone _____

Name _____ Telephone _____

These are other things that I would like to consider for
my labor and the birth of my baby:

_____

_____

_____

_____

_____

_____

✦ *DOULAS* ✦

Doula is an ancient Greek word. Of all the translations I've read my favorite is "walking with woman." It has a nice comforting sound to it, like having someone special in your life to care for you when you're in need.

Besides being a godsend you can trust at the most difficult time in your baby's life, a doula also brings loving comfort to a pregnant family. Many doulas have had babies themselves. Their own birthing experience, coupled with professional training, equips them to provide understanding, insight, and comfort to the laboring family. They often have an extensive library with plenty of information to share. They can refer their clients to classes, teach techniques for labor and the birth, and help moms adjust to their body's changes. Whatever else you call her—labor assistant, birth guide, midwife assistant, labor coach—a doula supports, educates, comforts, and provides spiritual, physical, emotional, and psychological guidance to the birthing family.

> Support, according to the Cochrane Collaboration's Pregnancy and Childbirth Group of Oxford, England, is essential for mothers in labor and "should include continuous presence, the provision of hands-on comfort and encouragement."
>
> The Group states that since there are "clear benefits and no known risks associated with intrapartum support," we should do everything we can to be sure that these mothers "receive support … from specially trained caregivers."
>
> Sure sounds like a doula to me.

What Does a Doula Do?

During pregnancy: The doula visits the pregnant couple at least two to three times before the birth. Together they put together a birth plan, rehearse various breathing and relaxation techniques, discuss labor, and decide when they should transport the mom to the hospital if she hasn't chosen a homebirth.

During labor and birth: A doula usually arrives at the couple's home soon after the onset of labor and evaluates the laboring mom. She helps the couple establish a rhythm that will maintain a steady and progressive labor. She's there as an addition to, not a replacement for, the mom's partner. She helps the mom stay at home as long as it's safe to do so, guides her with relaxation, provides food and fluids, and helps her get some rest or sleep. She quietly and consistently assesses the mom's labor. As mom progresses into the active phase of labor, the doula helps transport her to the hospital if that's the mom's choice.

In the hospital the doula provides ongoing support. She helps communicate the couple's needs and choices to the hospital staff. She helps interpret medical issues and procedures for the couple, and if decisions must be made, she explains the available options. But even though the doula is the couple's advocate and support, she never makes decisions for them.

Although the couple may feel they're strangers in a strange land, their doula is not. During their labor and birth, the doula is a constant. Even when shifts change and doctors, nurses, and midwives go home, the doula stays. She speaks up for the couple when conflicts occur. The experienced doula is aware of what is normal in the labor room, which in itself helps ease anxiety. She reassures mom about her progress and supports the birthing couple's wishes expressed in their birth plan.

The doula helping in a homebirth is a gift. During the mother's pregnancy she'll begin teaching breathing and relaxation techniques, she'll help her fix her home to accommodate the new arrival, will show her what she'll need to prepare for the big day, and will be available to her for any questions she may have. The doula will come when the mother starts labor—maybe even before the midwife—so she can labor with her and keep her comfortable. She'll prepare meals for siblings, make phone calls to have them watched, and make sure that the mother and partner don't have to deal with anything but their labor. The doula, if she has lots of homebirth experience, can be a second pair of hands for the midwife when moms give birth, and after the birth will help clean up and settle the mom and her partner and family to bed. She may come back every day for about a week to help the mom with breastfeeding and answer any questions she may have about her health and her baby. At a homebirth a doula is a must—a very welcome person to add to your circle of support.

The doula knows how to keep the mom physically comfortable. She can offer massage and help position the mom, and immediately after birth she can help with the bonding between mother and child and with breastfeeding.

> Research shows that a doula's presence facilitates several significant factors in labor and birth:
>
> ✦ A 25% reduction in the length of labor
>
> ✦ A 60% reduction in epidural requests
>
> ✦ A 30% reduction in analgesia use
>
> ✦ A 50% reduction in cesarean rate
>
> ✦ A 40% reduction in Pitocin use

The doula is also there for non-coaching fathers, siblings, and any other family members who may be present. She uses her loving and caring nature to ease anxiety and fear. She takes pressure off the dad so he can participate according to his own comfort level—and some dads feel very relieved knowing someone else is there for their partner. In general, the doula's many levels of care go a long way in keeping the environment calm for the mom.

During the postpartum period: Many doulas also provide postpartum care. One of their skills is to be able to teach the mom the fine art of breastfeeding. Your doula is most likely a mother herself with breastfeeding experience. She should have attended lectures, read a lot, and gone to conferences that taught women how to teach others breastfeeding without difficulty. She usually has a long list of books that she can recommend and may have a huge lending library at your disposal.

They have plenty of tricks in their bag that will make the postpartum experience easier and more successful. Some doulas even take care of household chores such as cooking, cleaning, running errands, laundry, or caring for the baby's siblings. This gives the mom and dad a chance to bond with their newborn and, just as important, allows mom and baby to rest and recover from the exciting birth experience.

Summary: So there she is—a woman's servant like no other. After a successful birth that included loving care from a doula, moms experience greater self esteem and have lower incidences of postpartum depression. Facilitating successful births with happy babies, moms, and dads is what a doula is all about.

Hiring a Doula

Now that you've read about the benefits of having a doula on your birth team and have decided to use one, you'll need to know how to find someone who's a good match for you. With the help of various resources, a computer, and the websites I've listed at the back of the book, you'll be on your way to hiring your own special advocate.

Of course you'll want to look in your own area first. Word of mouth is a basic and effective tool; get the word out that you're looking. Health food stores and herb shops may have bulletin boards with information about local doulas, midwives, and childbirth educators. Check your phone book. If it doesn't include a section that lists doulas, try calling some of the midwives, childbirth educators, massage therapists, or hypnotherapists that are listed and tell them what you're looking for.

Consider checking with your local mother/baby stores. One such store in San Francisco actually keeps current listings of various care providers. Try asking other mothers-to-be in your prenatal classes, your prenatal instructor, and your physician or the attending RN in the office. This will also give you an idea if your doctor supports the use of a doula, which will be very important to the management of your birth.

If a local search doesn't pan out, there's always the computer. You'll find that several organizations can not only help you locate a doula, but also offer birth and postpartum doula training courses if you decide to become one.

I have listed many doula search-sites in the Website section at the back of this book, but some of my favorites are:

Doulas of North America (DONA) — This is a nonprofit organization to train birth and postpartum doulas. Its membership to date includes 3,700 trained doulas, and you can use DONA's website to locate some of the doulas who are practicing in your area. *www.dona.org*

Childbirth and Postpartum Professional Association (CAPPA) — This international organization trains, certifies, and supports doulas, childbirth educators, and lactation consultants. They have an excellent doula search function listed by state. *www.childbirthprofessional.com*

Birthpartners — This organization's website is very user friendly and will help you locate a doula, midwife, childbirth educator, or lactation consultant in any area you specify. When you choose a doula, the site offers a short description of her services as well as her phone number and address. *www.birthpartners.com*

Midwifery Today — This organization has a website for locating a midwife, doula, or childbirth educator plus all kinds of information about the childbearing year. It also offers information about midwifery training. *www.midwiferytoday.com*

I'm confident that these sites will help you get your search started. But before you begin to contact the doulas you're interested in, be sure you're clear about the qualities that are important to you. Communicate what you're expecting from a doula and ask a lot of questions. You may want to interview several women before you make a decision. But after you do decide, be sure to call the others and tell them. Doulas can only accept so many clients a month, and knowing that you have chosen someone else will free them to make other commitments.

In her thesis "Doulas, Social Support, and Postpartum Depressive Symptoms," Laura Marie Wittman tells us that "postpartum depression affects not only the new mother, but her baby, her marital relationship, and her family and friends," so it is essential that we find services to help women "transition into motherhood." She says that study seems to indicate that women are helped by support geared to "a unique experience and transition in their lives." Further, she states that it is essential that we, as a society, find out all we can about easing that transition by "developing preventative measures" to fight the "negative effects of postpartum depression, because mothering is the most common occupation in the world, responsible for shaping the lives of future generations."

What to Ask

Like any important person you hire in your life, you want to know all you can about them. This is especially true when hiring a doula to care for you and your baby prior to, during, and after your baby's birth. Below, I have included some questions and why you should be asking them. Read them over and, using the worksheet at the end of this chapter, get them answered and written down. Let the results help you choose the right doula for you and your new family.

What training have you had?

There are many different types of doulas. Some are self-trained, and some have trained under another doula, read a lot of material, attended lots of births, and may even teach prenatal classes. This is similar to the concept of the direct entry midwives and sometimes not a bad thing. But be sure you get references, check how many births they've attended, and find out what they actually know and if they can handle an emergency situation.

Other doulas are trained through organizations like DONA (Doulas of North America), Midwest Doula Trainers, MotherLove, Inc., and several others. They take a very extensive training course, are given specific material to read and tests to take, and receive actual hands-on experiences to complete their training session. They have the backup of their organization and have people they can call if they have questions.

What is your experience with birth?

Experience is the best way to become a professional in this field. You can read, you can attend conferences, and you can talk with other doulas, but you need the hands-on experience to be good and reliable. Ask for references and talk to others who have used the doula you are considering.

What is your philosophy about childbirth?

This is important. What does your potential doula believe in and what are her priorities? What does she feel strongly about concerning your pregnancy, labor, and your baby's birth?

May we meet to discuss our birth plans and your role?

Is the person you're considering interested in your birth plan? Does she want to meet at least 2 to 3 times before you go into labor? Does she have ideas of her own and is she clear in explaining to you what her role is in your birth? Does she teach prenatal classes? What is her style of labor coaching? Does she know how to help you with the style that you're considering?

May we call you with questions before and after the birth?

Is your potential doula available 24/7? Does she have a cell phone or a pager? Can you call her and ask questions before you go into labor? Is she going to be available after you have your baby? For how long? Will she charge extra to be available after you have your baby?

When do you join us in labor? At home or in the hospital?

Will your doula come to your home while you're in labor? Does she have the ability to do cervical checks to see how far you're dilated before you go into the hospital? Is she only available to you after you enter the hospital? Will she stay throughout the whole labor and way past the birth? How long will she be there with you after you have your baby?

Do you have backup? May we meet them?

If your doula can't make it to the birth who will? When can you meet her? Does she have the same philosophy as the doula you originally hired? Is she going to charge a different fee? An additional fee? Does she know the hospital you'll be going to or the midwife you'll be using for a homebirth? Is she available 24/7 also?

Do you have references that we can call?

Can you get the phone numbers of at least four or five women she has attended? How about the hospital she has worked in? Can you talk to the physician about the doula you're considering and see if she knows about her?

What is your fee?

What does it cover? Will she take payments, or does she want the money all up front? Do you pay for her babysitter or gas? If you need postpartum care what is her fee for that?

Conclusion

This should get you started—don't be afraid to ask questions. If she is responsible and respected she won't feel offended and she'll be willing to give you phone numbers and any information or references you need. Choosing a doula to help you during your childbearing year may be the most important decision you'll make regarding your birth. I guarantee that when you find that special someone you'll create memories that will last a lifetime.

Hiring a Doula

Hiring a doula is different than hiring a physician or a midwife. A doula will be with you no matter what style of birth you decide on. She is a presence in the hospital and clinic, and at your home. She is the special someone who will be your labor coach; your breastfeeding advocate; your keeper of the siblings, husband, and friends; and in some cases she may even be the one who catches your baby. You'll have a deep relationship with your doula and you'll learn to trust her and lean on her during your pregnancy, labor, and maybe even weeks after.

Finding one takes some research. You can't usually find her in the phone book—you'll have to rely on other mothers who have hired one, hospitals, health food store postings, and the Internet. In the website section of this book are some sites that will show you where you can start your search.

So, get out your pencil and get ready to circle or check your answers and fill in the blanks. Start by making a list of potential candidates:

Name _____

Telephone _____

Address _____

_____

Years of Experience _____

References _____

Name _____

Telephone _____

Address _____

_____

Years of Experience _____

References _____

Name _____

Telephone _____

Address _____

_____

Years of Experience _____

References _____

Name _____

Telephone _____

Address _____

_____

Years of Experience _____

References _____

Interviewing a Doula

		Yes	No

1. What training have you had?
   DONA WORKSHOP
   _____

2. How many years have you been a doula? _____

3. Who taught you?

   _____

   Her phone number. _____

4. How many births have you attended? _____

5. What were your duties at these births?
   Emotional & Educational Support

6. Do you conduct cervical exams?   ☐   ☑

7. Have you caught any babies?   ☐   ☐

   If so, how many and why did you do the catching?

   _____

8. What is your philosophy of birth?
   a safe, normal presence, calmness

9. How many times do you visit before labor? *as needed*

10. Will you go over my birth plan with me?   ☑   ☐

11. Do you come to my home during labor?   ☑   ☐

12. Do you just meet us at the hospital? *unless you want*   ☐   ☑

13. Who is your backup if you can't make it?

    _____

    What is her phone number?

    _____

Yes No

14. What does she charge if she has to attend? _____

15. Can we meet her before I go into labor? ☒ ☐

16. Are you available for questions after the birth? ☒ ☐

17. Who are your references (and their phone numbers)?

_____

_____

_____

18. What is your fee? ½ on second visit, the other ½ after birth

19. How do expect to be paid? Cash, Check

During My Pregnancy

During your pregnancy you'll want your doula to help you in several different ways. Below are a few that you might want to jot down and present to her.

20. I'd like to take a prenatal class. ☐ ☐

21. I like to use following style for my breathing
and relaxation technique:

☐ Lamaze ☐ Bradley ☐ ICEA ☐ Local Hospital

☐ HypnoBirthing ☐ What my doula recommends

22. For my first and second trimester I'd like you
to recommend nutrition and exercise. ☐ ☐

23. During my third trimester I'd like you to prepare me
for my birth and tell me what to expect if I'm going into
the hospital, or how you'll help me if I'm having my
baby at home. ☐ ☐

24. I want you to teach me about breastfeeding. ☐ ☐

25. I need help with sibling care and managing
my home during my labor. ☐ ☐

26. When do you feel comfortable transporting me to the hospital (if I'm laboring there) and how will we go about doing this?

_____

_____

_____

From Labor through the Birth of Your Baby

	Yes	No

27. I'd like you to come over while I'm in early labor.   ❏   ❏

28. When you come, and if I don't need help with breathing or labor, I'd like you to:

   ❏ Prepare the siblings for the babysitter

   ❏ Prepare a meal for my husband

   ❏ Get my birthing room ready

   ❏ Just help me with my contractions

29. If you have the training, I'd like you to do cervical checks so we don't leave for the hospital too soon.   ❏   ❏

30. I'll probably need encouragement to keep moving and would like suggestions to keep my labor on track, such as:

   ❏ Bathtub   ❏ Walking outside

   ❏ Different positions   ❏ Massage

   ❏ Squats

31. When my contractions are steady at _____ minutes apart, and I can't talk through them, and if you're able to check me, and I'm at least _____ cm dilated, I'd like to be transported.

(Note: First-time mothers usually progress slower and can pretty much wait until the last minute, but women who have had other babies should not wait until they are dilated beyond 7 centimeters or are experiencing steady contractions that are closer than 5 minutes apart.)

	Yes	No
32. In the hospital, I want you to take responsibility for my birth plan.	❏	❏
33. I'll need you to interpret what the doctor is telling me about my progress.	❏	❏
34. I don't need any opinions or help with medical decisions. My partner and I will make all decisions.	❏	❏
35. I want to know how my labor is progressing and if I'm being told any half-truths.	❏	❏
36. If I need advice that's contrary to hospital routine, we'll discuss it in private and then tell the medical staff that your suggestions came from my partner— protecting you from any hard feelings.	❏	❏
37. If I have a cesarean and my partner doesn't want to attend, I'd like you to be there instead.	❏	❏
38. If my partner does attend my cesarean operation, I'd like you to be with my baby at all times.	❏	❏

After I Have My Baby

	Yes	No
39. After I give birth I'd like you to help me place my baby to my breast.	❏	❏
40. I'd like you to stay _____ hours after I give birth so my partner can take a short nap or run errands. I'd love your company and a chance to chat about the birth.	❏	❏

	Yes	No
41. I'd like you to help me for _____ days after I give birth.	❑	❑
42. I'd like to have your help with the siblings— preparing their meals, getting them off to school, after-school care, etc.	❑	❑
43. I'd like to hire you for postpartum care.	❑	❑
44. I'd like help with the baby at night for _____ days/weeks.		

Conclusion

Well that's about it. Your doula will be a good friend and a lot of help. She'll work hard to keep you on track with your labor, and can help you a lot after your baby is born.

If you have any other questions or concerns that I may have missed, include them below.

I wish you the best of luck with all the wonderful people that will be there for you on your special day. And please, please, please! Write me at Breck@writeme.com after you have your baby and tell me all about it. Promise?

Other questions I may want to ask:

_____

_____

_____

_____

_____

_____

_____

3
Medications
in Labor

◆

Sometimes Babies
Aren't All That's Being Pushed
In Hospitals.

"I've had enough of this doo-doo."
    —Peter, from *Three Men and a Baby*

D rugs, drugs, drugs. The moment you walk into a hospital in labor a nurse asks how painful your contractions are. You're asked to rate your level of discomfort and, if it's high enough, you're offered something to offset or alleviate the pain. The offer comes with a gentle reminder that there's no need to suffer. When you grimace during a contraction your partner is assured that you can be made more comfortable. So not only is the nurse offering you something, but now your partner is brought into the picture. At last convinced that you are indeed in unbearable pain and well aware that the remedy is at hand, you give in; you accept the pain medication. And things go downhill from there.

Most moms who take the time to understand childbirth and seek various options are interested in natural childbirth without medication. Nevertheless, if the labor becomes long or difficult and mom is overwhelmed or disheartened, she may request drugs. This doesn't mean she has failed at labor. There may be a time in labor where mom has had enough and wants help coping—it's a normal reaction and nothing to be ashamed of. However, mothers should know exactly how drugs can affect labor and baby.

> Each year more than one million Americans have to be hospitalized because of adverse drug reactions. These are drugs prescribed by conventional-medicine physicians.

Some hospitals don't understand or support the concept of natural childbirth, and their personnel encourage moms to use medication to ease labor, honestly believing they're helping the mother cope. Sometimes the reason is simple economics: costs in the medical community have risen to the extent that hospitals can't afford to employ enough staff for one-on-

one labor care. Keeping moms medicated or asleep with an epidural means a single nurse can care for several patients at once.

Nevertheless, avoiding the use of unnecessary pain medications is still possible. It's a matter of planning ahead and having a good support team on your side during labor and your baby's birth.

Following are some suggestions to help you keep on track and say no when you're offered drugs:

+ Hire a doula or professional labor support person who is experienced at labor management. Simply by having a professional support you through your contractions, you'll be surprised how well you do.

+ Exercise during your pregnancy. This strengthens your muscles and prepares your body for the long stress of labor. It'll also give you the endurance you need in case your labor is lengthy.

+ Consider a birth center or having a homebirth with a midwife. When you choose a setting other than a hospital, you're also hiring people who support your views.

+ Attend childbirth classes that teach non-pharmacological methods of pain relief such as yoga, HypnoBirthing, Lamaze, and others. If you're taught to think in terms of natural labor and birth, and practice that way of thinking and acting, you'll most likely go that route when the time comes.

+ In the hospital, ask the charge nurse on duty which nurse is the strongest supporter of natural childbirth, and ask that she be assigned to you. As a hospital-based labor and delivery nurse, I am surprised how many birthing styles the nurses have. Some avidly support the use of epidurals and Pitocin, and others bend over backward to keep the mom laboring naturally and spend extra hours keeping her comfortable and on track.

✦ Before considering pain medication, ask for a vaginal exam to see how far your cervix has dilated. You may be further along than you thought, and hearing this may encourage you to carry on without medication. I've seen newly admitted moms who are 3 or 4 centimeters dilated labor hard for an hour or so and then ask for an epidural or pain medication. But when I check them first, they have progressed to 7 or 8 centimeters. At this point they're only an hour or two away from being able to push.

If you still feel strongly that you need medicated pain management, these are your basic options: narcotic injection, IV, or epidural. (Many of the medications that hospitals used in the past are no longer available.) This chapter is intended to educate you about these options and how they will affect your labor and your baby.

✦ *NARCOTICS* ✦

Your provider can prescribe several different pain-reducing (not pain-relieving) medications. I've listed the most common here.

> **Agonist:** A drug that triggers a reaction, such as relaxation.
>
> **Antagonist:** A drug that blocks a reaction, such as pain.

✦ **Nubain** (nalbuphine hydrochloride) is a synthetic narcotic agonist-antagonist analgesic of the phenanthrene series. It's a potent drug that's equivalent to morphine. Its onset is about two to three minutes. Its use during labor can cause respiratory distress in the baby. This drug has numerous side effects and comes with many precautions for the mom and infant.

✦ **Butorphanol** (Stadol) has both narcotic agonist and antagonist properties. Analgesic potency is said to be as much as seven times that of morphine and thirty to forty times that of Meperidine, also known as Demerol. It is the most common drug given to laboring women, and it is safer then Nubain.

✦ **Fentanyl** (also called Sublimaze) is also a narcotic analgesic drug with numerous side effects for mom and especially for baby.

✦ **Demerol** and **morphine** have been around for a long time but are still commonly used during labor. Like the other medications already listed, each has adverse side effects.

Demerol stays in the system longest of the narcotics I have listed. When it's taken during labor it passes through the placenta to the baby. After the baby is born it will stay in his system for hours. If it's administered right before you have your baby, he may need aggressive interventions, such as oxygen and vigorous stimulation.

Morphine is usually given intravenously in small doses because it works fast and doesn't stay in the system as long. But again, if it's administered right before your baby's birth, it passes to the baby and results in a "floppy" infant at birth.

Effects on the Mother

The most common side effect of these narcotics is that they can slow down or stop labor if given too early. Sometimes when moms come into the hospital late at night with early labor, weak contractions, and haven't started dilating yet, providers prescribe morphine or Demerol in hopes of stopping the labor so the moms can rest. Usually after labor is slowed way down or stopped entirely they're sent home to sleep and instructed to come back when contractions are stronger and more effective.

For thirty minutes after a mom is given narcotics she must be placed on a fetal monitor to track the infant's heart rate. There are times when the baby doesn't tolerate the drug well, becoming sleepy and burdened by a heart rate that is dangerously low.

> Twilight sleep (a combination of morphine and scopolamine) was introduced into the United States in 1914. It became so popular that upper-class women formed "Twilight Sleep Societies," and obstetric anesthesia became a symbol of modern progress made possible through medicine.

Narcotics for pain management often only dull the pain slightly and make mom too sleepy to effectively deal with her contractions. Women often fall asleep between contractions, only to be startled awake in the middle of one, completely unprepared to control it with breathing techniques. She struggles through contractions with catch-up breathing, usually failing and falling back to sleep after the contraction passes. When her breathing techniques aren't working because her timing is off, she asks for more medication, convinced that the dosage was not enough to make the labor pain go away. The downward spiral begins at this point, and more and more interventions are needed to counteract the side effects of drug overload and to birth a healthy baby. This is called a *cascade of intervention*.

Narcotics may also cause nausea, and moms are often given another drug, Phenergan, to counteract it. This drug causes further drowsiness. Drowsiness in turn causes shallow breathing, which decreases the amount of oxygen mom delivers to her baby—which in turn decreases the baby's heart rate and puts the baby at risk.

Effects on the Baby

Narcotics easily pass through the placenta to the baby in undiluted doses and drastically affect the baby's heart rate, which can cause low blood pH and the baby to be floppy, blue, and in respiratory distress. Babies in these circumstances sometimes need aggressive intervention to keep them out of even more serious trouble. All drugs, including medicinal herbs, reach the baby, and any dosage that has an effect on the mother has the potential of having an overdosing effect on the baby, simply because the mother's body weight is about 20 times greater.

Narcotics administered late in labor undoubtedly affect the baby when he's born. A sleepy baby is difficult to rouse, may have problems keeping his heart rate up, may have trouble breathing, and may need to be admitted into the nursery for observation. These babies usually are too drowsy to latch onto the breast, missing an opportunity critical to establishing a good breastfeeding pattern. Drugged babies may also miss the important moments immediately after birth when they bond with their mother—making eye contact, breathing in mom's smells, and realizing they're being touched and cuddled. Instead, overdosed babies are placed on a hard surface—chilled because they're wet—suction tubing is forced into their mouths, their backs are vigorously rubbed, and cold oxygen is blown on their face to pink them up. Sometimes an oxygen mask is placed on their face and air forced into the lungs to initiate breathing. This is not a good way to come into the world.

And the medication didn't even take care of the discomfort of labor as mom had expected it would.

But awful as it sounds, narcotics are better than epidurals. Narcotics involve a shot in the hip or intravenous access and, when they're given after labor is well established, they don't slow labor down or impede pushing. You can move around easily, because after 30 minutes the monitor is removed allowing you to go the bathroom or stretch your legs. You'll be able to experience labor, and it may even help a little with back pain.

> "Prevention is a worthy and good cause. The problem is that her cousin, intervention, likes to follow only a few paces behind."
>
> —Mayri Sagady, CNM, MSN, and director of the UCSD Nurse-Midwifery Service in San Diego

✦ *EPIDURALS* ✦

Epidurals are all the rage for pain management. In fact, their use is epidemic. At some hospitals epidurals are offered the minute a laboring woman walks through the door. The number of laboring women given intrapartum epidural analgesia is reported to be more than 50 percent at many institutions in the United States. One major Pacific Northwest hospital offers epidurals right up to the moment moms are pushing. Their epidural rate is 98 percent, and some moms specifically choose this hospital on the advice of their friends who "breezed through labor while sleeping the whole time."

What is an Epidural?

Epidural analgesia, which provides pain relief during labor, is given by injection into the epidural space between two lumbar vertebrae in the lower spine. If successful, the analgesia blocks pain impulses, causing numbness from the waist to the thighs, or even to the toes.

I've witnessed numerous births that included the use of epidurals. And yes, the mom breezed through the many hours of labor, mostly asleep. But on the fetal monitor I've watched the baby's heart rate drop into the 80s with every contraction (normal is between 120 and 180). A mom is immobilized by an epidural and usually ends up lying on her back for hours. This can cause the baby to slip into a posterior position or to lie on the umbilical cord, cutting off his oxygen supply. Or it may simply cause failure to progress—one of the most commonly cited reasons for cesarean section. Mother's blood pressure often drops, causing the baby's heart rate to drop, decreasing his oxygen.

A labor slowed by an epidural often leads to the use of Pitocin (a synthetic oxytocin) to encourage the uterus to contract (read more about Pitocin later in this chapter). Because mom isn't feeling her contractions anymore, the Pitocin dose can be aggressively increased, bringing the contractions to a level she'd never be able to tolerate if she wasn't medicated. The intensity and frequency of the contractions are extremely stressful to the baby. The physical pressure on the baby is very hard for him to tolerate. The baby's heart rate may drop, increasing the risk of an emergency cesarean section.

An Epidural Story

One of the moms whose labor I attended as a doula, and who planned to birth her baby in the hospital, was having a picture-perfect labor at home. When we arrived at the hospital, however, her labor stalled. Although her weakened contractions continued, she was stuck at 7 centimeters dilation for an hour and a half. (Stalled labor commonly occurs when a mother is brought into the hospital—the body is being cautious and tries to ensure its safety after the cozy nest at home has been abandoned.) After she was admitted her nurse convinced her she needed an epidural to help her relax, get a good rest, and continue dilating. She warned that without it, if mom continued to labor without dilating, a cesarean would have to be performed because of failure to progress.

Soon after the epidural was administered the mom's contractions stopped, her provider was notified, and Pitocin was started. As a complication of one or the other (or both), the mother's blood pressure bottomed out, and the fetal heart rate dropped into the 60s, which is dangerously low. With emergency procedures and additional medication the problems were remedied and the mom was tucked into bed to sleep. It took nine more hours of labor for this mom to dilate the last 3 centimeters, with the baby's heart rate dropping into the 90s or 80s at every contraction.

The most maddening part of the whole episode was the hospital's adamant opposition to giving her a couple of hours to dilate naturally when she first arrived. My effectiveness as an advocate for the couple's wishes was at a serious disadvantage because the hospital staff had been lobbying to ban doulas from the labor and delivery ward. During the night, when the baby's heart rate was dropping into the 80s, I suggested that the doctor be notified. Staff responded that he didn't want to be disturbed until 6:00 a.m. When I voiced concern about the baby's heart rate dropping repeatedly, they assured the parents that everything was under control. When I questioned the unusually high Pitocin dosage, they told the parents that steps had been taken to balance it. When I told them they were all a bunch of quacks... Well, you get the picture.

> So common is the use of epidurals that many childbirth professionals are calling the 1980s and '90s the age of the "epidural epidemic." Eighty percent of the women in a study by Sargent and Stark received epidurals or their equivalent.

This baby was pulled out with forceps. He was floppy, blue, and beyond exhaustion. Apgar scores (a 0–to–10 scoring system, with 10 being best, used to evaluate the baby's condition after birth) were recorded. By my analysis as a neonatal intensive care nurse, the baby's scores were 3 at one minute and 5 at five minutes. The attending nurse rated him 8 at one minute and 9 at five minutes. I was appalled. Recording a high score on the baby's medical record, however, ensured that there could be no legal repercussions if the baby's protracted low heart rate during labor had led to further problems.

The 'Kim James' Version of Epidurals

A wonderful woman who has created a useful and balanced website to inform mothers-to-be about epidurals has granted me permission to pass on the following information. Thanks to Kim James, BA, CD (PALS), CCE (CEAS). Her web page address is *www.kimjames.net*. Please take time to visit it—you'll learn a lot.

Maternal Risks and/or Side Effects of Epidural Anesthesia

Most women will experience some side effects. Fortunately, the majority of these women will experience only the more annoying effects rather than the more serious.

Hypotension (drop in blood pressure)

How often it happens:

+ It's the most commonly occurring risk: 30 to 35 percent of epidural use.[1,2]

Why it's a problem:

+ Mother's blood pressure must be maintained at sufficient levels to assure oxygenation of the fetal blood.

+ Reduces blood supply to the placenta; baby is distressed.

+ At-risk babies may not have the reserves to handle even a small drop in the mother's blood pressure.

+ Maternal and fetal respiratory distress may develop.

What can be done:

+ To help prevent epidural-induced hypotension, you'll receive 1 to 2 liters of IV saline before the epidural is placed. You may also be asked to lie on your left side.

+ Ephedrine may also be given through the IV to restore blood pressure. You may also be given more IV saline fluid.

✦ Stay off your back. Compression of the abdominal aorta and the inferior vena cava may decrease uterine arterial pressure and increase uterine venous pressure.

Urinary Retention, Postpartum Bladder Dysfunction

Virtually all women will be given a urinary catheter to prevent urine retention and bladder distention during labor.

How often it happens:

✦ 25 to 34 percent will have bladder dysfunction after childbirth. [3,4]

Why it's a problem:

✦ It increases the risk of urinary tract infection.

✦ A full bladder inhibits dilation of the cervix and rotation of the baby's head.

✦ Bladder control may be lost for days, weeks, or months because of strain on numbed pelvic floor muscles.

What can be done:

✦ A nurse will insert a urinary catheter to drain your bladder.

✦ Choose a CSE (Combined Spinal Epidural), inserted through an intrathecal catheter in your back, so that you are more likely to feel the need to urinate and may also go to the bathroom yourself if hospital policy allows. Be sure a light dose is given; this could be strong enough that you'll feel nothing from the waist down.

✦ Practice pelvic floor exercises (Kegels) before and after childbirth.

Uncontrollable Shivering

How often it happens:

+ Frequent.[5]

Why it's a problem:

+ Uncomfortable for mother.

What can be done:

+ Use blankets, heat sources, and massage to relieve shivering.

Itching of the Face, Neck, and Throat

How often it happens:

+ Common.[6]

Why it's a problem:

+ More common with CSE epidurals because of the narcotics used.

+ More of a nuisance than a serious medical problem.

What can be done:

+ Women may be given a drug to combat the itching, which may have side effects of its own.

Nausea/Vomiting

How often it happens:

+ Common.[7]

Why it's a problem:

+ Uncomfortable for mother, but it usually lasts for only a short time (approximately 30 minutes).

+ Vomiting can waste needed resources and deplete mother's energy.

What can be done:

+ Medicine may be given to treat nausea. This medication sometimes makes the mother intensely sleepy.

Postpartum Backache

How often it happens:

+ 10 to 22 percent of the time. [8,9]

Why it's a problem:

+ Backache may last only a few days or may continue for years. It may be caused by "stressed" positions in labor exacerbated by muscular relaxation and the absence of feedback pain to tell you to get out of a damaging position.

+ May be the result of nerve damage (rare).

What can be done:

+ Change positions frequently.

+ Stay off your back.

+ Practice pelvic- and back-strengthening exercises to prepare for childbirth.

+ Consider choosing a CSE, or intrathecal epidural, to allow you more sensation and to avoid awkward positions.

Maternal Fever

How often it happens:

+ 15 percent of the time if the epidural is in place longer than four hours. The percentage increases the longer an epidural is in place. [10]

Why it's a problem:

+ Epidural anesthesia affects your ability to sweat. If you can't sweat, it's more difficult to dissipate excess body heat.

+ Uncomfortable for mother.

+ Baby's heart rate may become distressed from mother's fever, increasing the odds of having a cesarean section.

+ Babies are often separated from their mothers immediately after birth to check for infection. This exam may include a spinal tap to check for sepsis. Baby may stay in the hospital for several days for antibiotic treatment while mother goes home.

What can be done:

✦ Do not accept epidural anesthesia before active labor is established (dilation to 5 centimeters or more).

✦ Try to keep cool. Eat ice chips or drink ice water; keep ice packs under arms, under belly, or between legs.

✦ Have a birth attendant mist and fan you during labor to promote heat dissipation.

Spinal Headache

How often it happens:

✦ 1 to 10 percent of the time.[11]

Why it's a problem:

✦ A spinal headache is most likely caused by postdural puncture and cerebrospinal fluid leakage. It can range from mild to debilitating and last from days to weeks.

What can be done:

✦ Rest at home in a supine position (on your back).

✦ Drink caffeinated beverages, with the approval of your care provider.

✦ May resolve on its own, or you may need a blood patch procedure.

Uneven, Incomplete, or Nonexistent Pain Relief

How often it happens:

✦ 10 percent of the time.[12,13,14]

Why it's a problem:

✦ Some mothers find incomplete, inconsistent pain relief to be just as stressful as no pain relief at all.

What can be done:

✦ Talk to your care provider if you have inadequate pain relief.

✦ Epidural can be reinserted for better placement or the needle moved.

Feelings of Emotional Detachment

How often it happens:

✦ Depends on the mother.

Why it's a problem:

✦ Some mothers report feeling "detached" from the experience of childbirth as a result of the full effects of epidural anesthesia. Some mothers may not feel like participants in their births.

✦ May affect mother-baby bonding.

What can be done:

✦ Talk to your care provider and get new-parent support.

Postpartum Feelings of Regret or Loss of Autonomy

How often it happens:

✦ Depends on the mother.

Why it's a problem:

✦ Mother may have felt pressured to have an epidural anesthesia or regrets her decision. Mother may not have been well supported or respected during her labor.

What can be done:

✦ Talk to your care provider and get new-parent support.

Inability to Move About Freely on Your Own

How often it happens:

✦ 100% of the time.

Why it's a problem:

✦ Limited movement inhibits labor progress.

✦ It's boring, annoying, and discouraging for some mothers.

✦ Increases likelihood of cascade of interventions.

What can be done:

✦ Talk to your care provider about your concerns.

✦ Wait until you are at least 5 centimeters dilated before you request an epidural.

✦ Exhaust all other comfort measures before requesting an epidural.

Loss of Perineal Sensation and Sexual Function[15]

How often it happens:

✦ Unknown.

Why it's a problem:

✦ Most likely a result of forceps use and episiotomy, but it may also result from nerve damage.

What can be done:

✦ Talk to your care provider about any degree of sexual dysfunction after childbirth. This aftereffect is not normal, and options exist for correcting perineal pain. There may be no treatment for nerve damage, however.

Very Serious Risks of Epidural Use

✦ convulsions

✦ respiratory paralysis

✦ cardiac arrest

✦ allergic shock

✦ nerve injury

✦ maternal death

How often it happens:

✦ Extremely rare, ranging from 1 in 3,000 to 1 in 500,000. [16]

Baby Risks and/or Side Effects of Epidural Anesthesia

Epidural anesthesia is "generally regarded as safe" by the Food and Drug Administration. Though studies suggest that epidural agents don't harm the baby very much, no research proves that these anesthetic and narcotics don't harm the baby at all. No drug has ever conclusively been proven safe for a baby in the womb.

Fetal Distress, Abnormal Fetal Heart Rate[17,18]

How often it happens:

+ Unknown.

Why it's a problem:

+ Probably a secondary side effect of the epidural.

+ Fetal distress is most likely caused by a drop in maternal blood pressure or an awkward maternal position.

+ Increases the likelihood of an operative birth (forceps, vacuum, or C-section).

What can be done:

+ Get off your back or change positions immediately.

+ You may be given oxygen to help oxygenate your placental blood.

Drowsiness at Birth, Poor Sucking Reflex[19,20]

How often it happens:

+ Unknown.

Why it's a problem:

+ Interferes with mother-baby bonding immediately after birth.

+ Can be extremely frustrating for mothers trying to learn to breastfeed. Mothers may be encouraged to formula feed just to "get something into the baby."

What can be done:

✦ Remain with your baby. Let your baby sleep at your breast or next to you in bed.

✦ Try talking and singing to your baby.

✦ Refuse artificial nipples or supplemental formula.

Poor Muscle Strength and Tone in the First Hours[21,22]

How often it happens:

✦ Unknown.

Why it's a problem:

✦ Greater chance baby and mother will be separated immediately after birth. Baby may go to neonatal nursery for observation and oxygen.

✦ May be caused by lack of adrenaline from mother.

What can be done:

✦ Request that your baby stay in your room for all newborn procedures and observations, if policy allows.

✦ You or your partner go with the baby to the nursery and ask to hold the baby during all newborn procedures and testing.

Labor Risks and/or Side Effects of Epidural Use

The following side effects are often more common than maternal risks.

Prolonged First Stage of Labor

How often it happens:

✦ Common. [23]

Why it's a problem:

✦ The anesthetic in epidurals weakens all the muscles below the epidural site. This can dampen the strength of uterine contractions.

✦ Can be exhausting, boring, or otherwise discouraging for both mother and father.

✦ Increased use of Pitocin to strengthen contractions can be stressful on baby and/or the uterus, which may lead to cesarean section.

✦ Greater incidence of maternal fever.

What can be done:

✦ Give labor time to happen. Risks increase the longer Pitocin and epidural anesthesia are in your system. As long as mother and baby are doing well, allow time for labor to work. Do not accept arbitrary time limits. There is no "magic amount of time" for labor to be finished.

✦ Ask your nurse and care provider for reassurances that you and your baby are well.

✦ Negotiate with your care provider before labor happens how long you will be allowed to labor. Find out when your care provider will begin suggesting cesarean section for failure to progress.

Increased Incidence of Malpresentation of Baby's Head

Malpresentation is when a baby in utero or in labor is not presenting himself in the right position to properly descend through the birth canal. Descending feet first (breech), sideways (transverse), or face first (brow presentation) makes it very difficult to pass through the vagina without either causing a lot of tearing to the perineum, or getting the baby stuck in the birth canal requiring the use forceps or cesarean section.

How often it happens:

+ 20 to 26 percent of the time. [24]

Why it's a problem:

+ Relaxation of the pelvic diaphragm predisposes malpresentations, as do lack of mobility and inability to switch positions.

What can be done:

+ Choose a CSE or intrathecal epidural.

+ Wait until baby is very low in the pelvis (at least +1 or +2 station) before requesting an epidural.

+ Wait until at least 5 centimeters dilation before requesting an epidural.

Increases the Need for Pitocin Augmentation

How often it happens:

+ Almost always, especially if an epidural is given before five centimeters dilation. [25]

Why it's a problem:

+ Some babies simply do not tolerate Pitocin-induced contractions, the result being abnormal fetal heart rate after administration of the drug.

+ Abnormal fetal heart rate may necessitate an emergency cesarean.

+ Pitocin has many side effects (see "Epidurals and Pitocin" later in this chapter).

What can be done:

+ Wait until 5 centimeters dilation before requesting an epidural. If you give your body a chance to establish labor on its own, you're less likely to need augmentation.

+ Ask your care provider to wait at least two hours before Pitocin is started to give your body a chance to adjust to the epidural.

+ Your body must also process the IV fluids that were administered before the epidural. That much fluid very often dilutes the oxytocin in your body, resulting in weaker, more widely spaced contractions. Give your body a chance to process the excess IV fluid and catch up.

+ You may want to practice active visualizations in an effort to speed up your own oxytocin production.

Prolonged Second Stage of Labor

How often it happens:

+ Especially true for first-time mothers. [26]

Why it's a problem:

+ May go against some care providers' philosophy (e.g., second stage must be finished in two hours).

What can be done:

+ Wait to start pushing until the baby's head is visible on the perineum.

+ Negotiate with your care provider before labor begins how long you'll be allowed to push. Find out when your care provider will begin considering forceps, vacuum extraction, or cesarean section for failure to progress.

+ Change positions and use downward gravity to help push your baby out.

+ Stay off your back.

Decrease in the Ability to Push Effectively

How often this happens:

+ Common. [27]

Why it's a problem:

+ The buildup of anesthetic weakens muscles to the point of ineffectiveness.

+ Mother may be able to push a little, but may not be able to effectively help the baby rotate and descend.

+ Leads to increased likelihood of operative birth.

What can be done:

+ Stop pushing and wait until the contractions bring the baby's head down.

+ Shut off the epidural and wait for it to wear off so you will have the urge to push.

+ Change positions to see if this will help give you sensation to push.

+ Stay off your back.

Increased Likelihood of Forceps or Vacuum-Extraction Birth

How often it happens:

+ Five times greater likelihood. [28]

Why it's a problem:

+ Less efficient uterine contractions may keep baby from rotating naturally, and the diminished urge to push may keep baby from coming down.

+ Muscle weakness may not allow mother to push effectively.

What can be done:

+ Consider letting the epidural wear off for pushing.

✦ Don't request an epidural until you're at least 5 centimeters dilated. The fewer hours the epidural anesthesia is in your system, the less muscle weakness you'll have to contend with.

Increases the Likelihood of Episiotomy[29]

How often it happens:

✦ Depends on care provider's philosophy.

Why it's a problem:

✦ Goes hand in hand with increased use of forceps and vacuum extraction.

✦ Episiotomies are far more likely to tear beyond the original incision, making the opening larger then a natural tearing of the perineum and thus needing more repair and longer healing.

✦ Episiotomies take longer to heal and leave more scar tissue than natural tears.

✦ More postpartum pain for the mother.

What can be done:

✦ Talk to your care provider about his philosophy about episiotomies. Find out when he's most likely to do an episiotomy, and how often it happens in his practice.

✦ Strengthen your pelvic floor muscles before labor.

Increases the Likelihood of Cesarean Section

How often it happens:

✦ This is the likelihood you'll have a cesarean if you have an epidural dilated to the centimeters mentioned. Remember, you dilate from 1 to 10, then you are ready to push.

  — 50 percent of the time at 2 centimeters dilation.

  — 33 percent of the time at 3 centimeters dilation.

  — 26 percent of the time at 4 centimeters dilation.

  — After 5 centimeters there's no difference in the nonepidural group.[30, 31]

Why it's a problem:

✦ Cesarean section births carry far more risk to both the mother and baby than do vaginal births.

✦ Mother may feel cheated out of a vaginal birth experience.

✦ Postpartum recovery time is significantly longer than that of a vaginal birth.

What can be done:

✦ Don't request an epidural until at least 5 centimeters dilation. This'll give you the greatest opportunity to get labor established on your own and to be upright and active.

Here is a quick review of why an epidural is risky

◆ Slows down or even stops labor

◆ Increases the need for oxytocin to stimulate contractions

◆ May lead to a cesarean birth, especially for first-time moms

◆ Causes maternal fever, which can result in a septic workup or antibiotic treatments for the baby and a long nursery stay

◆ Anesthetics pass to the baby through the placenta

◆ Can cause significantly decreased heart rate in the baby and affect the baby's oxygenation prior to birth—which can interfere with breastfeeding

◆ May interfere with the rotation of the baby in early labor, thus interfering with descent and dilation—another reason for cesarean

◆ Can cause spinal headaches and respiratory distress in the mother

◆ Can cause life-threatening complications to both mother and baby

An epidural can offer these advantages:

◆ Can lower the blood pressure of a laboring woman who has pregnancy-induced high blood pressure

◆ Can help mom relax if she is very anxious, tense, and unable to handle contractions, making her labor lengthy and unbearable

◆ Useful if the mother needs a C-section; it's much better than using a general anesthetic

◆ Does not cause drowsiness or loss of sensation or muscle tone in upper extremities. Mom can turn easily and remain in some control of her labor

The Epidural Procedure

There is no such thing as a "quick fix" with epidurals. Administering one is a long, involved, complicated process. To begin with, an anesthesiologist must be located, which can take thirty minutes to an hour. In the meantime, a nurse starts an IV and free-flows a 500–1000 cc fluid bolus of either lactate Ringers or normal saline to help prevent the mother's blood pressure from dropping when the narcotic in the epidural is started. A fetal monitor is attached around her abdomen to closely track the baby's heart rate, and a blood pressure cuff is fitted on the mom's arm that will automatically inflate every fifteen minutes throughout her labor and her baby's birth. Because epidurals make mobility impossible and mom can't get up to go to the bathroom, a Foley catheter is inserted into her bladder to drain her urine. Meanwhile, forms are filled out, consents are signed, and the risks are explained.

When the anesthesiologist arrives, the procedure is explained and a medical history is taken. Mom assumes either a sitting or side-lying position on the edge of the bed. Remember that all the while the mother is contracting, she's being told she must be very, very still because he'll be looking over her back for the exact site where he'll be inserting the needle and catheter. While the anesthesiologist is preparing for the procedure, the nurse is helping the mother into position, breathing with her through her contractions, and attempting to keep her still. The anesthesiologist cleans the insertion area with Betadine, which will feel cold. He then numbs the epidural site with Lidocaine, places a needle into the epidural space, threads an epidural catheter (a thin plastic tube) through the needle, and then slowly removes the needle, leaving the catheter in place. The catheter and the tubing are taped to the mom's back. The anesthesiologist administers a test dose of analgesia to ensure there is no allergic reaction to the medication. If there isn't a reaction, he'll administer enough to make the mom comfortable. The epidural is hooked to a pump that administers a steady dose of medication that will, to varying degrees, numb the woman from the waist down. She'll have some sensation in her legs but they'll not be able to support her weight.

Ideally, patients will still be able to move their legs, but I've yet to see this be the case. Usually a mom feels nothing from the waist down, but to keep the medication from pooling in one area she'll need help moving from side to side every thirty minutes. Her blood pressure and heart rate must be recorded every fifteen minutes, and the fetal monitor will remain in use throughout the remainder of her labor. The doctor will probably order an internal fetal monitor, which requires that a small electronic probe be inserted through the cervix and gently screwed into the baby's scalp. And if that isn't enough, an intrauterine pressure catheter (IUPC) will be placed vaginally against the wall of the uterus to monitor the strength of contractions. Since the IUPC is a stiff plastic tube there is risk of puncturing the uterus while it is being inserted. For the internal monitor and the IUPC to be inserted, membranes must be ruptured. Hopefully, the umbilical cord won't slip past the head and create a prolapse—an emergency situation that calls for immediate cesarean section.

> **The Belly Dancer Alternative**
>
> Some cultures believed that belly dancing began as an ancient birthing ritual. Women of a village would dance around a friend in labor to help take her mind off the contractions.

✦ *EPIDURALS AND PITOCIN* ✦

Pitocin is synthetic oxytocin, the natural posterior pituitary hormone. The word oxytocin means "rapid birth." It stimulates uterine smooth muscle contractions indirectly and helps expedite the normal contractions of spontaneous labor. As in all significant uterine contractions, there is a transient reduction in uterine blood flow. In layman's terms, Pitocin is used to stimulate the contractions that the epidural stopped. It's almost a guarantee that if you're having an epidural you'll need some form of intervention to augment your labor, and it'll probably be Pitocin.

Pitocin is also commonly used to induce, or start, labor. Some providers rely on Pitocin to control labor so that a woman will have her baby before it gets too late at night and he's gone to bed (I'm not making this up). I feel the overuse of this drug is one of the biggest dangers for the laboring mom. It's interesting to know that in 1978 the FDA advisory committee removed its approval of Pitocin for the elective induction of labor. (The drug has never been approved by the FDA for the use of augmenting labor.) The current *Physicians' Desk Reference* clearly states that "Pitocin is not indicated for elective induction of labor." But it *is* used, constantly and almost always without the signed consent of the mother.

I'd like to make a comment here to confirm that yes, labor is going to hurt, cause cramping, can come on suddenly, and be very uncomfortable—*but it is manageable*. I think the horror stories you hear about overwhelming pain that needs strong and heavy-duty medications is induced by Pitocin. When your provider orders Pitocin the contractions are stronger, last longer, and are closer together (just like the doctor wants them) and the chances are you'll need something to ease the discomfort—and an epidural will usually be the most common request.

I think the most important thing I can teach you in this book is that there will never be a time during your labor when you can have just one intervention (like breaking your waters, stripping your membranes, starting you on Pitocin, giving you an epidural, keeping you on the monitor all the time, or giving you any type of pain medication). If you choose to have any of the above, it will almost invariably lead to other interventions (having to monitor your labor and baby more closely, giving you oxygen to keep the baby's heart rate up, birthing the baby with forceps or vacuum extraction, having a floppy baby, or keeping you from hemorrhaging after your baby's birth, for instance).

If an epidural is administered too early and your contractions start to peter out, your physician will order Pitocin to stimulate them. Pitocin is administered intravenously, with strict guidelines, with an infusion pump at a continuous and regulated rate. As you've learned by reading about the drug's adverse effects, you and your baby must be monitored very closely.

If all goes fairly well, your contractions will pick up again and you'll labor until you have your baby. However, Pitocin-induced contractions can become too intense, and the baby can start to show signs of distress. This is why your baby must be continuously monitored. Sadly, what makes epidurals so popular is that while you are laboring away with contractions that are stressing your baby you're feeling hardly any pain at all. The pain that you would be feeling from the intensity of the contractions would warn you that you are getting way too much Pitocin and would force the provider to cut down the dose. So, without the pain there is virtually no limit to how much Pitocin you could receive. This ends up being very comfortable for you, but very bad for your baby.

Birthing itself can go many different ways. If the epidural is shut off when the mom is 8 to 10 centimeters dilated, she may feel enough sensation to push her baby out. If not, then baby must be vacuum extracted or pulled out with forceps. Pushing can go on for a couple of hours, putting a lot of stress on the baby, and most likely mom will get a large episiotomy. If the epidural is started early, chances are 33 to 50 percent she will end up with a cesarean.[32, 33] After birth, the baby will likely be stressed and need help breathing and pinking up. Mom will be numb for the next hour or more. Breastfeeding is delayed, and for quite some time the baby can have neurological residuals or some numbness himself from the epidural.

Have a serious and in-depth talk about epidurals with your birth partner, and be sure you understand all the pros (few) and cons (many) for you and your baby. It's scary that parents are not properly informed about all the potential complications. Just as disturbing, moms who have already birthed using an epidural will—because of lack of education about its dangers—recommend it to anyone who'll listen. But it's not a safe method of pain management for either mother or baby. The risks almost always far outweigh the advantages.

A Guide to Effective Care in Pregnancy and Childbirth, published in 1995,[34] states that epidurals cause "well-established complications" that include low blood pressure, nausea and vomiting, prolonged labor, increased use of forceps, vacuum extractions, and cesarean sections. Breathing difficulties, nerve damage, and even maternal death can occur. It doesn't sound like a very safe choice to me.

Read *The Thinking Woman's Guide to a Better Birth* by Henci Goer. This is a well-researched and well-written book by a wonderful woman who is dedicated to revealing the truth about interventions. I insist that all my moms buy it—and read it!—when we first start working together.

Adverse effects of Pitocin include:

◆ Hypotension or hypertension

◆ Tachycardia (rapid heart rate)

◆ Dysrhythmia (uneven heart rate)

◆ Angina pectoris

◆ Anxiety

◆ Seizure

◆ Nausea and vomiting

◆ Allergic reaction

◆ Uterine rupture (from Pitocin-induced excessive contractions)

✦ *CYTOTEC* ✦
A Major Drug Warning

Okay, I've talked about epidurals, Pitocin, and narcotics, and pointed out their good points and their bad points. When used cautiously, responsibly, and for the right reasons, they might help a laboring mom.

But there is one drug that's becoming very popular but is *never okay to use at any time during your pregnancy or labor*. That drug is Cytotec.

Cytotec (or misoprostol) is a prescription drug that's used for certain stomach problems such as gastric ulcers. But because one of its side effects is severe cramps or contractions of the uterus, health care providers soon found that it induces labor so effectively that a birth was guaranteed within twelve hours of administration. But it's not a win/win situation. While the provider does get home in plenty of time for dinner, the mom is subjected to a very intense, ongoing labor with contractions occurring one on top of the other until her baby is born.

And then there's the warning label—a very clear, very adamant, and very serious caution that Searle (the manufacturer) puts on every bottle of Cytotec. It warns against the administration of Cytotec to pregnant women because it can cause abortion, premature birth, birth defects, maternal death, or uterine rupture (just to name a few potential problems). Searle even followed this up with a detailed warning letter that they sent to *all* health care providers in the United States (see the following page). It is also important to know that as this book goes to press, Cytotec has not been approved by the FDA for the use of inducing or augmenting labor.

August 23, 2000 --
Important drug warning concerning unapproved use of intravaginal or oral misoprostal in pregnant women for induction of labor or abortion.

Dear Health Care Provider:

The purpose of this letter is to remind you that Cytotec administration by any route is contraindicated in women who are pregnant because it can cause abortion. Cytotec is not approved for the induction of labor or abortion.

Cytotec is indicated for the prevention of NSAID (nonsteroidal anti-inflammatory drugs, including aspirin)-induced gastric ulcers in patients at high risk of complications from gastric ulcer, e.g., the elderly and patients with concomitant debilitating disease, as well as patients at high risk of developing gastric ulceration, such as patients with a history of ulcer.

The uterotonic effect of Cytotec is an inherent property of prostaglandin E1(PGE1), of which Cytotec is [a] stable, orally active, synthetic analog. Searle has become aware of some instances where Cytotec, outside of its approved indication, was used as a cervical ripening agent prior to termination of pregnancy, or for induction of labor, in spite of the specific contraindications to its use during pregnancy.

Serious adverse events reported following off-label use of Cytotec in pregnant women include maternal or fetal death; uterine hyperstimulation, rupture or perforation requiring uterine surgical repair, hysterectomy or salpingo-oophorectomy; amniotic fluid embolism; severe vaginal bleeding, retained placenta, shock, fetal bradycardia and pelvic pain.

Searle has not conducted research concerning the use of Cytotec for cervical ripening prior to termination of pregnancy or for induction of labor, nor does Searle intend to study or support these uses. Therefore, Searle is unable to provide complete risk information for Cytotec when it is used for such purposes. In addition to the known and unknown acute risks to the mother and fetus, the effect of Cytotec on the later growth, development and functional maturation of the child when Cytotec is used for induction of labor or cervical ripening has not been established.

Searle promotes the use of Cytotec only for its approved indication. Further information may be obtained by calling 1-800-323-4204.

Michael Cullen, MD
Medical Director, U.S.
Searle

Just think about it. If Searle is so aware of the risks and complications associated with Cytotec when it's used off-label (which means when it's not being used for what it was originally intended) that they are compelled to spend lots of time and money on all those letters, then you may be certain that this product is extremely dangerous and the death-cautions are very real to you and your baby.

But the scandal doesn't stop with just label warnings and letters. Ina May Gaskin wrote an article called *Cytotec: Dangerous Experiment or Panacea?* posted on Salon.com. In it she refers to approximately 20 studies of Cytotec-induced labors (1,958 births total). The results of these labors included two maternal deaths, 16 baby deaths, 19 uterine ruptures, and two hysterectomies. So according to these numbers, there's a 9.7% chance of a uterine rupture; compare this to the 0.3% chance of uterine rupture cited as the reason providers won't allow previous cesarean women to birth vaginally because the risk is too high! But even more scary, there's an 8% chance that your baby will die from complications and a 1% chance that you will.

Health care providers aren't blind—*they know all this*. And it's shocking! How can a provider, for the sake of his own convenience, one who took an oath to "do no harm," administer this unapproved drug to a laboring woman knowing full well that it will cause uncontrollable contractions and possibly kill her and her baby? No wonder malpractice insurance is so high.

I have seen providers "discretely" insert Cytotec vaginally during an exam without the mothers consent or knowledge. This is called "administering medication without a consent" and is illegal. So you must ask your provider if he uses Cytotec and, if he does, tell him that you won't allow it in your labor (preferably in writing). If he insists that it's safe and not all that dangerous, then run, don't walk, out of his office.

If you're still unsure and would like to read more, Dr. Marsden Wagner gave me permission to reprint his awesome article *Technology in Birth: First Do No Harm*. Dr. Wagner is a perinatologist, neonatologist, and perinatal epidemiologist, and is a consultant for the World Health Organization and UNICEF.

Thank you, Dr. Wagner, for the following article that clearly shows how a laboring woman (who at the time is in no position to argue) can be manipulated and put at risk by a provider for the sole reason of his own convenience.

Erratum: The decimal placement in 3 percentages in this paragraph is incorrect. They should read 0.97%, 0.8%, and 0.1% instead of 9.7%, 8% and 1%.

Technology in Birth: First Do No Harm
By Marsden Wagner, MD

Several years ago a drug with the generic name misoprostol (called Cytotec by the drug company that manufactures it) was approved by the Food and Drug Administration (FDA) as a prescription drug to be used for certain ailments of the stomach. It is known that one of its side effects is severe cramps or contractions of the uterus, and for this reason the label says it should never be used on pregnant women. Obstetricians, however, discovered that given orally or vaginally, Cytotec, because of its side effect of violent uterine cramping, can induce (start) or accelerate labor.

So without any prior testing of Cytotec for labor induction, obstetricians began to use it on their birthing women. Doctors on the Internet began to describe their experience with this new way of inducing labor. One doctor wrote, "I must say I have heard some great things about Cytotec myself. Just be careful. The stuff turns the cervix to complete mushie." A few studies have appeared in obstetric journals, but all the studies are too small to give adequate scientific evidence about this use of the drug. These studies did show some risks, such as a tendency for the fetus's heart to start racing, as well as other signs of fetal distress, and the explosion or rupture of the uterus in a few women. A review of the scientific evidence by a highly prestigious scientific body says that because of the lack of sufficient scientific evaluation and the reports of serious side effects, the use of Cytotec for labor induction "cannot be recommended for routine use at this stage."

The fact that Cytotec is not approved by the FDA for labor induction, is not approved for this use by the drug manufacturer (who still states on the label that it is not to be given to pregnant women), is not endorsed by either the American College of Obstetricians and Gynecologists or midwifery organizations, and is not approved by scientists for routine use, has had no apparent effect on the enthusiasm with which doctors are starting to use it. And there is nothing to stop doctors from using Cytotec for this "off label" purpose, because although the FDA must approve a drug before it goes on the market, once it is on the market for a specified purpose, any doctor can use it in any dose for any purpose on any patient.

After one obstetrician in South Dakota proudly told me over lunch that he was the first doctor in his community to use Cytotec for labor induction and now urges other doctors to use it, he justified his actions: "We will wait forever for the bureaucrats at the FDA in Washington, D.C., to approve drugs, so we must try them out ourselves if we want progress." When asked, he admitted he doesn't tell the women to whom he is giving Cytotec that the drug is not approved for this purpose, nor does he ask for informed consent. He scoffed at my suggestion that he is experimenting on women without their knowledge, much less their consent. The Oregon State Health Department told me their records show Cytotec to be the most common way of inducing labor in that state, and it is used on thousands of laboring women.

The use of Cytotec on birthing women has spread like wildfire for a very simple reason, told to me by many doctors: its use brings back the possibility of "daylight obstetrics" — that is, women brought to the hospital first thing in the morning and induced with Cytotec will give birth by late afternoon and the doctor can be home for dinner. How many women will have their uterus ruptured before a court case finally applies the brakes to this practice? I personally welcome learning of cases where Cytotec induction was used without fully informed consent and there was subsequent uterine rupture, cervical laceration or other serious complications.

The unsystematic, untested way in which Cytotec for labor induction was introduced and disseminated is typical for the technologies used during pregnancy and birth. Ultrasound scanning during pregnancy and electronic fetal monitoring during labor are further examples of uncontrolled introduction and dissemination of untested technologies. There is a big gap between what we know to be the best scientific maternity care practices and what is actually practiced. As a result, there is no consumer protection except litigation. Doctors blame lawyers and women for the fact that more than 70 percent of American obstetricians have been sued one or more times, but litigation is the only way a woman and her family can protect themselves against malpractice.

Many of the motivations behind the use of technologies by doctors are non-medical. Several examples, all supported by scientific study, will illustrate this fact. Studies of birth certificates show that birth is most common Monday through Friday, 9 a.m. to 5 p.m. The only explanation that can be given is that doctors and hospitals use the induction of labor for their own convenience. More shocking are data that show emergency cesarean sections to occur most commonly on weekdays during the daytime. Deciding to declare a labor an emergency situation requiring emergency surgery is influenced by the convenience of the staff.

Another non-medical factor that motivates the use of technology is money. Data from several states in the U.S. show cesarean sections to be least common among women on Medicaid and most common among private patients in private hospitals. One would think the opposite, assuming that poor women have poor health and need more interventions. But doctors and hospitals make bigger profits if technology is used in cases where the patients or their insurance can afford to pay. Commercial interests also play a role—manufacturers of drugs and technologies have a variety of ways to influence doctors to use their drugs and machines, including bestowing a wide range of gifts and perks.

Word Games

Providers are sometimes very disingenuous when they want to encourage you to accept a procedure or medication for a quick delivery. Below are a few that I myself have heard over and over again. And you know what? If you're not prepared with an informed answer they work every time to the advantage of the provider.

"You know, you've been laboring for quite a while now and your cervix is still only 'x' cm dilated. I think we should start you on Pitocin to 'kick start' your contractions and get this baby out."

Notice that this provider didn't suggest any natural solutions, like getting into a shower, walking, using a birth ball, or nipple stimulation. He just went right for the drugs.

Solution: If you feel you have a good relationship with your RN, talk to her (or better yet, your doula if you have one). Find out if your baby is in any trouble and have the RN go over the fetal heart rate pattern with you. Then ask yourself these questions: Is the baby doing okay? Are you getting the support you've wanted? Are there other things you can try besides drugs? If your answers are yes, then simply tell your provider, "No thank you, I'm doing just fine." It's no coincidence that a lot of medical interventions surface around 1 to 3 p.m.—just when the provider is trying to wrap-up his day.

"You've been at 'x' cm for the last couple of hours now. I don't think the baby is able to fit through your pelvis, so I'm recommending a cesarean to help this baby out."

This suggestion is not always the correct procedure. Sometimes it's presented to a laboring mother in the early evening when it looks like she may be delivering in the middle of the night. Some providers are not fond of coming back in the wee hours of the morning and will try anything to rush things along. Remember also that surgical teams are only in most hospitals during the day and they too hate to be called in the middle of the night for a birth if you really are having problems.

Solution: During your prenatal visits ask your provider, after scheduled ultrasounds, if he feels that your pelvis is adequate to deliver the size of baby you're having. Continue asking up to your very last visit. Then, if he suggests that the baby is too big for your pelvis, politely ask him how this could possibly be since *all* the ultrasounds proved that your baby and pelvis were a match. If he doesn't have a very adequate answer then tell him that you would like to get up and walk around, or take a shower or whirlpool bath, or use the birth ball to help bring your baby down. And then after that, you'd be willing to reevaluate the situation. But do keep in mind that he may be right, so talk to your RN after he leaves the room.

"Your baby is showing signs of stress. We need to perform a cesarean right away."

Solution: Ask to see the fetal monitor strip, have him show you where and when your baby was showing stress, and then ask to see the strip for over the last 15–20 minutes. See if there is any recent and ongoing stress or if it is an isolated incident that was resolved when you changed positions or moved the monitor pads. A lot of times a dip (or deceleration of heart rate) can happen when you're in a position that causes the baby's head to press his umbilical cord against something solid, like your spine or hip bone, which can cut off his oxygen supply and drop his heart rate. A simple fix for this is just a quick position change. Sometimes the heart rate does stay down for a short while, in which case oxygen is given to the mom along with the position change. If the heart rate of the baby returns to normal and **stays that way,** then the baby is out of danger. When this is the case, tell your provider that, as long as your baby is doing well, you'd rather continue laboring as you are, and that you want to get up, walk, sit on the birth ball, or shower. Remember, by not accepting an epidural, heavy pain medications, or Pitocin, you'll be able to get up and do these things. If you do accept an epidural then you're numb and immobile and this makes it much easier for the provider to manipulate you further.

"When I call the nurses' station in an hour I'd like you to be at 'x' cm or we'll have to start you on Pitocin."

If your provider can get you to accept a time limit on your laboring progress then he can use that when he inquires how you are doing and give orders to your RN saying that you have agreed to interventions.

Solution: Don't ever allow yourself to be placed on any time limit. Tell the provider that you'll labor at the rate your body is choosing as long as the baby is doing well, and that you'll let him know when you're ready to push—even if it's in the middle of the night.

"Do you want a dead baby?"

Believe it or not, I have actually heard this from a couple of providers after a mother has questioned their suggestions for interventions. Unfortunately it's very effective—what can you say?

Solution: Know your information. State that, No, you don't want a dead baby, and that's why you're refusing the risks involved with Pitocin, epidurals, and the 5–6 times higher risk of mortality and morbidity associated with cesareans. If you can rattle off a few risks and statistics with each intervention then the chances are good that your provider will back off and allow you to labor as you originally planned. Also be sure that your significant other knows this information. Having the father of the baby well informed helps a lot with your position to avoid drugs. Of course, if the individual characteristics of your problem dictate the use of medication in labor, this solution may be wrong for you.

Fortunately, not all providers are this deceitful and controlling, and I hope the one you've chosen isn't. But if you hear any of these statements or something similar, then please be on your toes—he may just want to be home for dinner.

Medications

My many years of experience in birthing and observation as an RN in maternity wards has brought out a strong personal passion against the use of drugs in labor. As you've read in this chapter, the practice has become epidemic and—in my opinion—obscene. Natural childbirth (one without the use of drugs) is now the rare exception rather than the norm. When a woman has her baby without medication everyone at the nurse's station gossips about it—words like "wow" and "amazing" are coupled with comments about it being "the first one this month!" I feel it's sad and appalling that the medical profession is indiscriminately pushing whatever drug comes to mind or whatever drug is currently in vogue to warrant such comments.

How to Help Prevent the Desire for Drugs

Check all that are important to you.

❏ Before I go into labor I'll take prenatal classes geared to natural childbirth.

❏ I'll hire a doula for labor management.

❏ I will enroll in a prenatal exercise class to strengthen my muscles in preparation for childbirth.

❏ I plan to hire a physician that uses midwives for labor coaching.

❏ I will look into additional classes that teach non-pharmacological methods such as HypnoBirthing, Yoga, Lamaze, etc.

❏ I will go to a birthing clinic instead of an OB/GYN for my prenatal care and birthing experience.

❏ I will only have people that are supportive of natural childbirth in attendance.

❏ I'll use other methods of pain management at home and in the hospital, such as the bathtub, the shower, breathing and relaxation, music, walking, and using my support persons for encouragement.

❏ In the hospital I'll ask the charge nurse to assign me an RN that supports natural childbirth and won't encourage the use of medication.

❏ Before accepting medication, I'll have my RN check how far I've dilated, and then make my decision. I'll not take pain medication before _____ cm or after _____ cm.

❏ I'll not accept a routine IV/heplock.

   If one is started it will be with the understanding that nothing will be placed in it without my approval and without complete justification for it. In other words, not just because "we do it with each delivery."

If I Do Use Medication

If you do agree to medication, there are things you need to ask yourself in order to get the most comfort with minimal side effects. But remember, after asking for that initial medication, it's very rare that it will be the only intervention you'll experience during your labor and your baby's birth.

❏ I will never allow the use of Cytotec in my labor. I know that there is no favorable research that proves this medication is safe in labor.

❏ Since I know that morphine is only 1/7 as potent as Stadol, and 1/30 to 1/40 less potent then Demerol, I'll start with morphine for pain management.

❏ I don't want the nurse to offer any medication until I ask for it.

❏ I'll ask her to start me on the lightest dose of pain medication to see how I handle it.

❏ I'll wait until my baby is very awake on the monitor and the heart rate is steady above 120 before taking medication.

❏ I will not take pain medication after 7 cm of labor because I know it will cause my baby to be sleepy when born.

❏ I'll avoid Demerol IM or IV because I know it is too potent.

❏ Because I know it will slow my labor, I don't want medication early in my labor—even if recommended by my care provider.

❏ If my labor is slowed due to medication, I do not want Pitocin to accelerate my contractions.

❏ If my labor slows, I want to first try nipple stimulation, reflexology, acupressure points, birth ball, and being mobile.

❏ I'll only consider an epidural as my last option of pain management.

❏ I'll wait until I am over _____ cm and my labor is well established before considering an epidural.

❏ I'll read again all the side effects of epidurals and other narcotics outlined in this chapter.

❏ I won't have Lidocaine injected to my perineum while I am pushing because it will cause swelling and increase the risk of a tear.

Refer to this completed worksheet when you write your birth plan. This will help you outline your desires in the use or refusal of drugs and let everyone concerned understand your choices and rights. I realize this looks like an awful lot of decisions to make, but this is the most crucial part of your laboring process. Read a lot, then research more. Weigh all options; take your own health into consideration—and the health of the baby you are carrying. And above all, don't be afraid to just say no to drugs. It's your body, your baby's body, and, legally as well as morally, these choices are all within your rights as a responsible, informed, patient and mom.

So you go, girl.

4

Herbs
in Pregnancy
and
Childbirth

◆

Mother Nature's Medicine Cabinet

"Nature does nothing uselessly."
    —Aristotle

Choosing alternatives to your birthing plans may also include choosing herbs. This is a personal choice and I'm including it in this book to help you get an idea of how herbs can help you throughout your pregnancy.

I've been using herbs along with conventional medicine for my health and the health of my family for most of my life. While I was practicing midwifery I routinely recommended several favorites to my pregnant moms. I also used them to help maintain my family's overall health. And even though my kids never got used to the taste or smell of some of them, they were still wonderful and effective supplements to the contents of my medicine cabinet.

When my youngest daughter was thirteen months old we found out, after all other procedures failed, that she needed surgery to repair a hole in one of the lower chambers of her heart. A few months before her scheduled open-heart surgery she contracted a staph infection during an overnight stay in the hospital. It settled into her lungs, giving her a chronic cough. Because of her heart condition she was diagnosed with

---

Important cautions

✦ Although the recipes, herbs and procedures described in this chapter are quite common (the information was gathered from websites and professionals around the U.S. and Canada) always consult with your midwife and/or physician before using them. As is true of any treatment, herbs can be dangerous when they're used unwisely or in excess—especially during pregnancy.

✦ Watch for allergic reactions. Always test new herbs and combinations in moderation until you're sure they don't cause any adverse reactions.

✦ Be careful to use correct doses—some herbs are much more potent than others.

✦ Always keep herbs fresh. Herbs like carbon dioxide, so put them in a plastic bag, then blow air into the bag as if it were a balloon, and seal it tight.

"failure to thrive," meaning she had stopped growing and would eventually die of malnutrition if her heart wasn't repaired. But the surgery was about to be cancelled because she couldn't risk it with such a severe infection. Canada's socialized medical system doesn't easily accommodate rescheduling, and she again would have been placed at the end of a six-month waiting list. We simply had to get rid of the infection.

During the next four months her doctors prescribed four different pharmaceutical antibiotics. Each time the doctors assured me that "this one will do it," and each time the antibiotic accomplished nothing. At last, I visited a local health food store owned by a client whose birth I had attended. She recommended Dr. Christopher's Anti-Plague syrup—a stinky garlic-based concoction. It was a struggle to get it down my daughter's throat three times a day. But it worked. Just six days later, with only two weeks to spare before the surgery, the infection was gone. And boy, did it ever feel great when I told the doctor that the stinky garlic-based herbal concoction had cured my daughter's infection! Her surgery was successful, and she is now a healthy twenty-six-year-old with boundless energy.

I later treated my other daughter's sore and swollen throat with herbs. Three months of antibiotics wasn't helping, but an echinacea-based spray destroyed the infection in less than one week.

Just as effectively, midwives use herbs to treat morning sickness and heartburn, diminish stretch marks, prevent miscarriages, tone the uterus, prepare women's bodies for breastfeeding, help them through labor, and much more.

In their natural form, herbs are just plant parts—leaves, flowers, roots, seeds, bark, and so forth—that must be prepared in certain ways before you can use them. You can buy practically anything readymade at a health food store, but it doesn't take much to prepare the herbs yourself, and it's actually quite fun. You may get a satisfying sense of involvement in the process of healing that you wouldn't otherwise get with a pharmacological treatment.

Common Methods of Preparation

Infusions

Infusion is a method of brewing herbs and using the extracts that are the end product of medicinal constituents in their flowers, leaves, and stems. Infusions aren't the same as teas. Infusions are made in the same way teas are made, but they're steeped longer so they're considerably stronger.

The standard recipe for most infusions is to pour a pint of boiling water over one-half to one ounce of dried herbs that have been placed in a quart jar. Seal the jar, steep the herbs for ten to twenty minutes, then strain and drink. When using fresh herbs, double their quantity.

There are other ways to prepare infusions. One way is to place the herbs in a glass jar, pour boiling water over them, seal tightly, and allow to steep overnight. Drain and drink in small portions. Another way is to place herbs—fresh or dried—in a pan, cover with cold water, seal with a tight-fitting lid, and bring the water to a boil over very low heat. Remove from the heat and let steep for about twenty minutes before using. Or place herbs in a jar with water, seal it, and set it in the sun until the infusion is the desired strength—usually all day.

Some people even maintain that herbs for feminine use (and for romance!) should be infused by the moon. When you infuse herbs using moonlight, the cooler temperature requires an open bowl and letting the mixture stand overnight. Drink first thing in the morning.

Infusions are taken in small doses—usually one to two teaspoons at a time, and up to one to four cups a day. Because of the time it takes to make infusions, they are usually consumed warm or close to room temperature. The biggest problem is their bitter taste—but think of the bitterness as nature's way of discouraging overdose. You may wish to add honey and/or lemon to make the taste tolerable.

Infusions have a short shelf life, so make them only as they're needed. It is best to steep the herbs in glass, enamel, or porcelain.

Decoctions

A decoction is a more aggressive method of water extraction for stubborn plant materials such as roots, bark, nuts, and non-aromatic seeds. Unlike infusing, which only requires simple steeping, decoction requires placing the herbs in boiling water, covering tightly, and then simmering over very low heat for fifteen to twenty minutes. Strain and drink while fresh.

A similar method is to place the roots, bark, nuts, or non-aromatic seeds in a pot of cold water and slowly bring to a simmer over low heat. Cover with a tight-fitting lid and simmer for fifteen to twenty minutes. Instead of straining and drinking the herbal mixture immediately after it's finished simmering, you could let it sit overnight for a stronger decoction that would maximize the properties of the herb.

Herbal Oils

Herbal oils aren't the same as essential oils you may have seen in stores, but instead are an easier type made using infusion. They are good for massage and ointments to treat conditions such as rashes, minor burns, cuts and stretch marks, and to act as insect repellants.

Choice herbs for making herbal oils include:

aloe vera	*lilac*
bergamot	*lime*
bitter almond	*meadowsweet*
caraway	*narcissus*
dill	*orange flower*
eucalyptus	*neroli oil*
fennel	*peppermint*
gardenia	*rose (attar)*
heliotrope	*rosemary*
honeysuckle	*rosewood*
jasmine	*sandalwood*
lavender	*tonka bean*
lemon	*vanilla*
lemon verbena	*wallflower*

I recommend using dried herbs because they're less likely to go rancid. But if you choose to use fresh herbs, keep bacteria from proliferating in the mixture by placing it in the sun for a day so all the moisture evaporates from it before using. Use only high-quality oils such as those extracted from seeds, nuts, or vegetables. Virgin olive oil is best for medicinal purposes, and grape seed, apricot kernel, almond, or canola oils are recommended for massage.

Place the herbs, dried or fresh, in a glass container and cover them with the oil of your choice to two inches above their surface so that when the herbs swell they won't be exposed to air. Seal the container tightly, set it in a sunny place, and let it infuse for two weeks.

Oven method: Place the sealed glass container of herbs and oil in a pan of water so it's half submerged. Set the oven to its lowest temperature and heat for a couple of hours, checking frequently to avoid burning. This method saves a lot of time if you need a particular herbal concoction in a hurry.

Crock-Pot method: Place the sealed glass container in a Crock-Pot set on the low temperature setting. Cover and heat two to four hours, as you would all your herbal oil methods.

Whichever method you choose to make your decoctions, when you're finished strain the herbal mixture thoroughly through cheesecloth or muslin and store it in glass jars, tightly sealed, in a cool, dark place.

Tinctures

A tincture is an herbal preparation made in alcohol or liquid glycerin using dried or fresh herbs. The best tinctures require high-quality herbs—fresh or dried—and pure grain alcohol such as 80- to 100-proof vodka. If you want alcohol-free tinctures you can use distilled water or white vinegar. (Don't use rubbing or wood alcohol, which are poison.) You'll need a glass jar with a tight lid, cheesecloth, labels, and a dark storage area.

Now this may sound a little "out there," but to add natural drawing power to their tincture, some people believe they should start the process during a new moon so that after two weeks it will be ready during a full moon. To prepare a tincture, put finely chopped herbs in a glass bottle or jar and cover them with vodka or liquid glycerin (or distilled water or white vinegar for alcohol-free tinctures). Seal the container, place it in a cool dry area, and let it sit for about two weeks, shaking the container at the same time every day. Strain the tincture through cheesecloth into a clean jar, preferably one that is amber colored or wrapped with brown paper to keep light from penetrating the glass. Squeeze the cheesecloth hard to get all the extract from the herbs. Store the tincture in a capped container in a dark place. Be sure to label the tincture with the names of the herbs you used, the day you processed it, whether it is a new- or full-moon preparation, what alcohol you used and how much or what proof, and for what purpose you are making the tincture. Tinctures can keep for up to ten years.

A tincture is used by either placing drops of it under the tongue or by diluting it in a favorite drink. The usual dose is approximately one teaspoonful taken three times a day. Tinctures can also be used in compresses, and for massages by placing a few drops in virgin olive oil.

Salves

Salves are made by heating an herbal oil of your choice (make the herbal oil as previously directed and wait two weeks until it is ready), adding beeswax to it, and melting them together to create a salve or cream. For each cup of your strained herbal oil concoction, add one-quarter cup of beeswax. Using a double boiler to avoid scorching, slowly melt them together. When the combination is melted, test the consistency by placing a small amount in a glass jar and putting it in the freezer for about five minutes. This should harden it to the consistency it will be when it's ready. If it's too runny, slowly heat the solution and add more wax. If it's too thick, add more oil and slowly heat and mix. After you have tested it using the freezer method and it is the consistency you want, remove the final batch from the heat and pour into small jars. Store the jars in a cool dark place. The salve should keep for several months.

Herbs to be Avoided in Pregnancy

Before I introduce some wonderful herbal remedies to help you through your pregnancy, I want you to know which herbs shouldn't be used during pregnancy. <u>CAUTION</u>: Some of these herbs may cause abortions, so familiarize yourself with their names. Read the labels on herbal preparations carefully to make sure these herbs aren't part of the preparations.

Avoid these herbs during pregnancy:

Blue cohosh

Black cohosh

Barberry

Cottonroot

Dong quai

Goldenseal:

    Limit your intake to
no more than one-quarter
teaspoonful per day.

Ginseng

Ginger, except in small amounts

Horsetail

Hyssop

Licorice

Motherwort

Myrrh

Mugwort

Mistletoe

Mandrake

Pennyroyal

Parsley

Rue

Squaw vine

Sage

Sarsaparilla

Shepherd's purse

Tansy

Yarrow

Some herbs are also contraindicated when you are breastfeeding. The herbs in the following list with an * next to their name may cause your milk supply to diminish or dry up.

Aloe vera

Basil

Black cohosh

Bladderwrack

Borage

Bugleweed

Cascara sagrada

Coltsfoot

Comfrey

Elecampane

Ephedra

Foxglove

Imitation vanilla

Licorice

Nightshade

Parsley*

Sage*

Senna

Wormwood

✦ *HERBAL TEAS* ✦

There are some wonderful herbal teas that you should start drinking as soon as you know you're pregnant. Replace your morning coffee and daytime sodas with these teas. Several of my favorites are described below, and I've included some recipes to treat various conditions. I'll start with the favorites first:

Red Raspberry Leaf

Red raspberry leaf is the safest herbal tea for the pregnant mom. It is superb for toning the uterus and the muscles of the pelvic region. It's rich in vitamins—particularly C and E—and contains calcium, iron, phosphorous, and potassium. It has a bit of an earthy taste that some people tone down by adding honey. To make the tea, add one heaping teaspoon of dried leaf to a tea ball, place it in a cup, pour boiling water over it, let it steep for fifteen to twenty minutes, and strain if necessary. Icing the tea is also great. Drink a couple of cups a day.

The benefits of red raspberry leaf tea are legendary:

- ✦ It tones the uterus and helps prevent miscarriage and postpartum hemorrhages.

- ✦ It helps relieve morning sickness throughout the pregnancy.

- ✦ By toning the muscles of the uterus and pelvic region it helps control the pain associated with uterine stretching and cervical dilation during labor.

- ✦ It helps produce and enriches breast milk.

- ✦ It helps relieve the discomfort of uterine cramping after birth when baby is breastfeeding.

- ✦ It helps alleviate the leg cramps during your pregnancy that could be caused by low levels of calcium and potassium in your system. Raspberry leaves contain both of these minerals.

- ✦ It relieves constipation and diarrhea.

Nettle Leaves

Nettle leaves are very rich in minerals and vitamins. They're high in iron, calcium, and folic acid, and contain more chlorophyll then any other herb. This herb has all the vitamins, plus potassium, phosphorous, and sulfur. It's also notably rich in vitamin K, so be sure to drink plenty of this tea, particularly in the last month of your pregnancy, to ensure good blood clotting when you have your baby.

As with raspberry tea, add a heaping teaspoon to a tea ball, place it in a cup, pour boiling water over it, and let it steep for twenty minutes before drinking. If you get tired of nettle tea and still want to get the nutritional benefits, the fresh leaves can be lightly steamed and eaten like spinach.

Some of the benefits of nettles are:

✦ toning the kidneys—nettle infusions have been known to loosen and dissolve kidney stones

✦ providing all the major vitamins and minerals to mother and baby

✦ relieving fluid retention

✦ helping prevent varicose veins and hemorrhoids easing leg cramps

✦ preventing hemorrhage (because it contains an impressive amount of vitamin K)

✦ increasing the quantity and richness of breast milk

Alfalfa Leaves

Alfalfa contains many essential nutrients, including some minerals. The most important nutrient is vitamin K, which is necessary for blood clotting. This is a good tea to drink during your last trimester to help you:

✦ decrease the risk of postpartum bleeding or hemorrhage

✦ increase breast milk production

Chamomile Leaves

Chamomile, a calming tea, is good for many of the common discomforts of pregnancy. It's frequently used in Europe as a treatment for nausea and to ease digestion. <u>CAUTION</u>: During pregnancy, however, limit your intake to one cup per day because it is a mild emmenagogue, which promotes the menstrual flow and could cause a miscarriage.

Chamomile is known to:

+ help alleviate insomnia
+ relieve heartburn
+ add calcium to the diet
+ help alleviate constipation

Dandelion Root and Leaves

Dandelion, which can be taken as a tea or as fresh leaves added to salads or sandwiches, is high in vitamin A, iron, calcium, and potassium. Some of its best-known properties include:

+ digestive aid
+ mild diuretic that helps reduce swelling of hands and feet
+ mild pick-me-up for times when you have less energy
+ blood pressure reduction when taken in combination with garlic oil capsules
+ liver cleanser and toner

✦ *HERBAL REMEDIES* ✦

Now you know about some of the best teas to drink throughout pregnancy to help keep you healthy. Doubtless there will be times when you're sidelined with a common pregnancy-related discomfort or two. This section includes some herbal remedies to help offset them.

Nausea of Pregnancy

Morning sickness (which, by the way, can happen any time of the day) is probably the number-one complaint of newly-pregnant moms. Morning sickness, which isn't to be confused with hyperemesis gravidarum, a more severe version of pregnancy-induced nausea, usually begins in the first trimester and (with any luck) will pass by the time you're in your second. Some moms find it sufficient to simply eat soda crackers before getting up in the morning to settle their tummy. Others don't have it quite that easy, but starting the day with a cup of herbal tea may help calm the stomach.

Ginger is widely known to help settle stomachs, but it mustn't be used in excess. Drink no more than one cup in the morning as your daily quota. You can sip ginger tea, take ginger capsules, or keep gingersnap cookies by your bed to snack on before getting up.

Ginger Tea Variations:

✦ Add one to two teaspoons of fresh ginger root to water, bring to a boil, and simmer for a few minutes. Add honey or lemon to taste. This tea can help alleviate vomiting.

✦ Place a blend of one to two teaspoons of ginger root and one teaspoon of fresh peppermint leaves in a cup, add hot water, and let steep for ten minutes.

✦ Mix one part raspberry and peach leaf mixture to two parts peppermint and one-half part grated ginger root. Add one quart cold water, heat to simmer, and infuse for twenty minutes.

Black horehound in tincture form can help prevent vomiting. Add one-half teaspoon to one cup of hot water and sip two to three times a day.

German chamomile reduces the feeling of nausea and calms the stomach.

It can be taken in tincture form—five to ten drops in hot water—or as an infusion, one cup before getting out of bed in the morning. Do not exceed this amount per day.

If you are susceptible to morning sickness, avoid strong smells that can bring on nausea. Try eliminating wheat or dairy products from your diet for the first couple of months—sometimes the stomach just can't handle those kinds of foods. A vitamin B6 deficiency could also be the culprit. Either try a vitamin supplement or add yogurt, bee pollen, nutritional yeast (great on popcorn), egg yolk, or organ meats to your diet. Also try using a heating pad on your tummy before getting up in the morning.

Ask your doula for recommendations. Most likely she'll have some wonderful ideas that have proved successful for her other moms.

Heartburn

Heartburn is caused by an overproduction of digestive acids and usually occurs during the last two or three weeks of pregnancy. The best way to avoid it is to eat small, frequent meals, chew your food slowly, and not take a lot of liquid with your food. Stay away from sweets, citrus fruits, and cheeses. Even though you may feel like lying down, it will only make heartburn worse, as will sitting hunched up or bending over.

Papaya is a terrific natural remedy. It can be taken in tablet form, as a tea, or as fresh fruit.

Slippery elm throat lozenges sometimes work as a quick fix.

Several herb teas help relieve heartburn. Peppermint is the one I recommend most often, but rosemary, chamomile, fennel, and lemon balm are also effective. Ask your doula what she suggests; she may know of other herbs that work well for her clients.

Umboshi plums can help offset heartburn. Eat the fruit, then suck on the seed.

A doula I know says this recipe works great for her moms.

Combine:

+ two parts fennel seed
+ three parts peppermint
+ two parts anise seed
+ one-eighth part lavender
+ one part cinnamon

Add two to three tablespoons of the combined herbs to a pint of water and bring to a boil. Remove from heat, cover, and let infuse for fifteen to twenty minutes. Strain and drink in small amounts throughout the day.

The following herbal combination also can relieve heartburn. Make a tea of equal parts of:

✦ meadowsweet

✦ dandelion leaf

✦ chamomile

Steep for fifteen minutes, strain, and drink.

Essential oils, which are naturally-occurring pure oils obtained from the distillation of a plant, can help when rubbed on the abdomen. Try:

✦ fennel

✦ lemon balm

✦ rose

Stretch Marks

Stretch marks are tiny tears in the second layer of skin that occur when it's stretched beyond what is normal. This stretching breaks down the elastin and collagen fibers and causes stretch marks, loss of tone, fine lines, wrinkles, and scarring. The scarring can vary in color from dark purple to light pink. Culprits are rapid weight gain, heredity, body building—and pregnancy.

But take heart—these little marks can be prevented, or at the very least they can be made less obvious. Best of all, the remedy involves lots and lots of massages. Oils and lotions applied to your skin penetrate the top layer and help repair damage to the second layer.

Stretch marks usually occur on the breasts, abdomen, and thighs because these areas expand the fastest during pregnancy. The key to preventing the scars from forming in the first place is to keep your skin moist and elastic. Just a few minutes of care each day will make a world of difference in how well your skin accommodates all the expanding.

When you first notice that these areas are growing larger, immediately begin applying massage oils at least once—preferably twice—a day. The most effective oils are coconut, olive, wheat germ, almond and, of course, the all-important vitamin E. Cocoa butter works nicely too. Drinking lots of water also helps keep your skin moist and pliable.

My moms have had great success with a weekly routine of two days of castor oil to break down the scar tissue, two days of olive oil to re-nourish the skin, and two more days of wheat germ oil to help rebuild tissue. Apply morning and night. On the seventh day use nothing. This will also fade a fresh cesarean section scar in only six months and an older scar in about one year.

Following are a couple of midwife-approved recipes to treat stretch marks. They are sweet smelling, and you'll love pampering yourself with them.

Recipe One

Blend:

+ Three parts coconut oil

+ One-half part beeswax

+ One part cocoa butter

+ One part vitamin E oil

Put all ingredients in a pan and heat on low until melted. Place in a small glass container with a lid and let cool before applying. The beeswax keeps the contents in a salve-like form and makes it easier to apply. Apply twice a day to the areas you're most concerned about.

Recipe Two

In a dark five-milliliter bottle, combine:
+ five milliliters of wheat germ oil

+ twenty drops of almond oil

+ twenty drops of lavender oil

+ five drops of nerotic oil

Blend by shaking container.

Massage over your breasts, hips, thighs, and belly in the morning and before retiring at night.

Early in your last trimester, begin to regularly massage oil around your vagina and perineum to promote stretching when you are having your baby.

Hemorrhoids

Hemorrhoids are varicose veins of the rectum. In women they are usually associated with pregnancy. These veins, which are internal and/or external, become enlarged from the pressure of your baby and straining when you have a bowel movement. Unfortunately, they are often painful and can sometimes bleed, although they're usually not dangerous or life threatening. Common symptoms are bright-red bleeding, painful swelling of the anus, and itching. During pregnancy, hormonal changes, taking iron tablets, and not ingesting enough fiber often causes constipation, which aggravates or even causes hemorrhoids. Keeping your stools soft and having a movement every day will help prevent them.

You can help prevent hemorrhoids by:

+ getting regular exercise
+ adding plenty of fruits and veggies to your diet
+ avoiding straining while having a bowel movement
+ drinking lots of water

You can relieve the discomfort and shorten the duration of hemorrhoids by:

+ placing ice packs on the affected area
+ keeping the anal area clean
+ sitting on a special "donut" cushion
+ applying lemon juice or witch hazel to reduce swelling
+ taking herbal sitz baths. Some good herbs to use are comfrey leaf, yarrow, marshmallow root, calendula, and a little sea salt. *Great Mothers*™ sitz bath formula is a wonderful product to try for postpartum relief. Her website is *www.greatmothergoods.com.* Check out her website.
+ applying baking soda, wet or dry
+ avoiding standing for long periods of time
+ avoiding heavy lifting
+ elevating your legs as much as possible during the day
+ applying an ointment made with comfrey or yellow dock root

Use the following mixture as a cold compress for comfort and healing. Combine in a small jar:

✦ one part witch hazel

✦ one part glycerol

✦ one part rose water

Apply with a cold cotton cloth three times a day.

Cold compresses of any type will help increase circulation and reduce pain and swelling. If nothing else, apply cold witch hazel.

Do not diagnose hemorrhoids yourself. See a doctor if you have rectal bleeding or pain.

Threatened Miscarriage

Threatened miscarriage is defined as any unexplained bleeding during the first twenty-four weeks of pregnancy. Although this occurrence can lead to an actual miscarriage or spontaneous abortion, it often doesn't. Some bleeding just happens; it could be the time of month you usually had your period, it could mean that during sex your cervix was abraded, or it could happen for no reason at all. About half the pregnancies that include some bleeding continue to term, and the babies are born healthy.

As tragic as they are, some miscarriages are bound to happen. Often, it's nature's way of ending a pregnancy that wasn't developing well. According to the National Library of Medicine, most early miscarriages (as many as 60% of first trimester ones) will remain unexplained. It is usually assumed these losses are genetic, where the chromosomes simply didn't replicate correctly. Over half of all miscarriages are caused by chromosomal factors that can cause a fertilized egg to die and slough off; this is completely out of our hands. These types of miscarriages aren't preventable—there's nothing we can do to stop them from happening, and they only rarely happen again. A poorly formed placenta or umbilical cord, a hormone problem, or a health condition we didn't know about can also cause miscarriage—and miscarriage may be the best outcome in the long run.

Other threatened miscarriages can be prevented with no risk to mom or baby. A cervix that's too relaxed and opens early in pregnancy, called an *incompetent cervix,* or an irregularly shaped uterus, can be remedied using various medical procedures.

Other miscarriages can be caused by infection, maternal age over forty, chronic disease, or accidents, and some causes will just never be known.

Some threatened miscarriages are caused by stress, trauma, inadequate diet, or weak uterine muscles. Herbs have been known to help prevent threatened miscarriages when they're used in conjunction with proper medical attention. But before I begin to discuss them, I want to share some common-sense, rule of thumb healthcare measures you can use to help minimize the risk of miscarriage. *Of course, before you use herbal or other treatments if you think you are miscarrying, consult with your doctor.*

Watch your diet. Many good prenatal books include a section about nutrition, and your childbirth educator or doula can also advise you about how to nourish yourself optimally to reduce the risk of miscarriage. The most basic guidelines include avoiding excessive use of caffeine (remember that cola and other soft drinks, most commercial teas, and, unfortunately, chocolate, contain caffeine) and eliminating tobacco, alcohol, and drug use altogether. Handling raw meat can cause toxoplasmosis, so use rubber gloves or wash your hands well after touching raw meat. And while you're pregnant please make especially sure that all meat is well cooked.

Avoid Stress. Eliminate as much stress from your daily routine as possible. Look into learning some yoga practices if you haven't already — it's a wonderful form of stress management and exercise. Your blood pressure will be a good indicator of how well your body is handling your pregnancy. Take your blood pressure periodically, and if it's ever over 140/ 90 inform your doctor — he may want to do follow-up work. (Some supermarkets provide free access to blood pressure monitors.)

Exercise. Exercising during pregnancy can improve your posture, relieve back pain, strengthen muscles in preparation for labor, enhance circulation, and increase energy. Many prenatal exercise programs are now available, and your doula will probably be able to recommend some.

If you think you may be miscarrying, call your midwife or doctor immediately. Some definite signs of miscarriage include:

+ light to strong cramps that can cause you to double over with pain

+ heavy bleeding that soaks a pad in a few hours or less

+ passage of tissue, such as a large clot

Slight bleeding and small darting cramps are usually normal indications that your uterus is stretching and pulling to make room for the baby growing inside you. Following are some herbal remedies that will help calm the uterus and offer extra nourishment and strength. But always call your provider when any bleeding occurs.

One doula recommends using a tincture made from:

+ three parts cramp bark
+ one part false unicorn root
+ one part black haw

If you think you're experiencing a threatened miscarriage (spotting and slight cramping), add one-half teaspoon of this tincture to one-quarter cup of warm tea and drink every half hour. This herbal tincture quiets the uterine muscles and eases the tension that often precipitates uterine contractions. But again, call your provider if you have any bleeding, no matter how slight it is.

For painless bleeding, mix two tablespoons each of:

+ black haw
+ false unicorn root

Place the herbs in a quart of boiling water and let the tea simmer for thirty minutes. Remove it from the heat and add:

+ one tablespoon blue cohosh
+ one tablespoon red raspberry

Strain and drink one cup every two to four hours until the cramping and bleeding have stopped.

For spotting or light bleeding, a doula friend recommends mixing:

+ one part raspberry leaf
+ two parts shepherd's purse
+ one part nettle leaf

Add the herbs to a quart jar, pour boiling water over them, and let steep for twenty minutes. Drink one-quarter cup every half-hour as soon as you see any bleeding; continue until the bleeding stops.

Another formula that works well is the following combination of tinctures and dried herbs.

First make an infusion of tea from:

+ one tablespoon cramp bark

+ three tablespoons raspberry leaf

Place the infusion in a quart jar, top with boiling water, and let steep for about twenty minutes. Then add:

+ eight drops wild yam tincture (contains hormonal precursors to cortisone and progesterone that help maintain pregnancy)

+ eight drops false unicorn root tincture

Drink about one cup every three to four hours.

Remember, whenever you feel your pregnancy is threatened, call your physician immediately. The teas and tinctures I have described are good measures to use immediately and continue using until you see your doctor.

✦ *AN HERBAL POTPOURRI* ✦

Over the years I've collected helpful information about herbal treatments from doulas and midwives across the country. It's wonderful to know that so many birth partners are using herbs in their practices. Herbs have been used for thousands of years to ease childbirth, stimulate mom's milk flow, and keep mom calm and feeling well. They're regularly prescribed by midwives, childbirth educators, physicians, doulas, and birth partners. Read through this selection, choose which herbs you think are right for you, and review your findings with your birth partner.

A doula from California says,

"The most commonly used herb, and one that I used through my own pregnancies, is raspberry leaf tea at least once a day. This herb helps tone the uterus and I have seen some very short labors for women who have used it faithfully. Used all across Europe, China, and North America, red raspberry leaf is rich in vitamins B, C, and E, and is very rich in iron, calcium, potassium, and phosphorus. The high fragerine content in the leaves strengthens the uterus and tones the pelvic muscles, giving you an easier labor and birth by making the uterus more effective. If you do nothing else with herb teas, drink at least two or three cups of this tea each day."

A New York midwife says,

> "Raspberry leaf has been used as a fertility tea for both men and women. It can help relieve morning sickness and can be used to help alleviate postpartum bleeding. Ask your doula for raspberry leaf tea combinations she likes to use. I bet you will be amazed how much she uses it in her practice."

A Canadian practitioner writes,

> "Tinctures that are good for calming nerves and promoting sleep are basil (also really good for morning sickness), catnip (great for insomnia), oatstraw (a wonderful nerve tonic), chamomile (great for nerves and keeping calm and focused), and lobelia."

A prenatal instructor from Florida offers these words of advice:

> "For heavy bleeding with periods and for postpartum bleeding try shepherd's purse or yarrow in tincture form. These aren't as aggressive as Pitocin, and you can administer them yourself after your midwife or doula leaves. Tinctures of ironweed and chamomile are good for menstrual cramping. Both of these can be placed in tea or under the tongue."

A practitioner from Washington advises,

> "For indigestion of any kind use a tincture of yellow root or slippery elm bark added to peppermint or ginger tea."

A Wisconsin lactation consultant says,

> "To promote an ample supply of breast milk, I recommend fennel seed, nettle, and raspberry leaf teas taken regularly while breastfeeding. If for any reason you need to decrease the flow of milk, use sage."

Another lactation consultant suggested blessed thistle tea for enriching and promoting breast milk. Combine:

- ✦ one part blessed thistle
- ✦ two parts nettle
- ✦ four parts fennel seed
- ✦ two parts raspberry leaf

Place about six tablespoons of this mixture in one quart of cold water. Slowly bring to a boil over low heat. Remove from heat and let infuse for fifteen to twenty minutes. Drink at least three cups a day.

This bit of information comes from Manitoba:

> "Nettles are an excellent source of iron, vitamins C and A, and calcium and protein. It has a strong diuretic effect and is good for treating edema. It helps lower blood sugar and tones the liver and kidneys. Strong infusions of this herb can help stop postpartum hemorrhage as well."

A doula in New Orleans says,

> "For labor contractions that aren't very effective or to help induce labor, try blue and black cohosh. CAUTION *This is a very potent herb and must never be used in early pregnancy because it can cause contractions.*"

From Oregon comes this advice:

> "For a postdate mom, mix ten drops of blue cohosh in one ounce of water; drink an ounce every eight hours if the baby is ready to be born—her labor will start. Blue and black cohosh are hormone balancers and will help the mom keep on track with her contractions so they don't phase out. Use oils of ginger, valerian, and lavender, and massage over the stomach and back to strengthen the contractions on a prolonged labor. CAUTION *Don't use before your due date because these herbs may cause contractions to begin.*"

An RN from Montana writes,

> "For perineal healing, comfrey leaves work wonders. Mash the leaves into a pulp; add vitamin E oil and honey to make it stick. Apply it to the perineum and cover with a peri-pad. Or it can be boiled down, strained, and placed in a plastic bottle. Pour onto the perineum when voiding to soothe and heal. It's also a great herb to add to a sitz bath, and drinking cold comfrey tea right after birth works well to prevent postpartum hemorrhage."

Check out the book reference section in the back of this book where I've listed some great herbal books for you to explore. The section also lists websites that offer information about herbs that can be beneficial during your pregnancy and childbirth.

IMPORTANT: Be sure to consult your physician if you're interested in using herbs, especially if you intend to correct a condition. The condition may require interventions other than herbs. Ask lots of questions, visit your local health food store, and relax with a soothing cup of peppermint tea.

How about a quick shopping list for teas:

_____ red raspberry leaves

_____ nettle leaves

_____ alfalfa leaves

_____ chamomile leaves

_____ dandelion root and leaves

_____ ginger root

_____ peppermint leaves

_____ black horehound

_____ German chamomile leaves

_____ slippery elm leaves

These are handy to have around the house when you are looking for a soothing refreshment while reading.

5

Complementary Methods of Pregnancy and Labor Management

✦

*Reflexology
and Hypnobirthing
and Yoga...
Oh My Again!*

"Cherish forever what makes you unique, 'cuz you're really a yawn if it goes."
—Bette Midler

We no longer have to enter a hospital in labor and use just one method for breathing or have to rely on medications for pain management. In the last 20 years, as laboring parents we've come a long way and now we have several choices on how to manage our baby's birth.

As you read in the previous chapter, more and more pregnant women are using herbs to help with discomforts such as morning sickness, stretch marks, or breastfeeding. (Ironically, women were using these herbs hundreds of years ago.) But that's just the beginning. We can also use yoga for our prenatal exercises, HypnoBirthing for breathing and relaxation, and reflexology and acupressure for pain management. Techniques that were only offered to a few previously are now available to us through specially trained women who can teach us how to make our pregnancy and birthing manageable. It's so exciting to see all the new information that's available now! We can endlessly explore on the Internet, looking for other options for childbirth and acting on them by contacting other pregnant parents who are also looking for choices. We can email each other across the country and tap into all kinds of resources that will make our birthing experience special.

These next few sections will give you an introduction—only an introduction—to some of these other options. You'll need to consult with a specialist on each subject for more in-depth information and special training.

✦ *HYPNOBIRTHING*® ✦

One of the greatest strengths of a birth professional is her ability to coach moms through their surges, helping them to keep calm and focused on their task of birthing their baby. It's an art of tried and true techniques that are as different as are the parents, with success stories for all. But one new technique that I'm hearing about over and over again is HypnoBirthing.

> Special thanks to Mickey Mongan, the founder of **HypnoBirthing**®, for allowing me to use material from her website.

The founder of HypnoBirthing®, and author of the book *HypnoBirthing—A Celebration of Life*, is Marie (Mickey) Mongan, M.Ed., M.Hy, of Concord, New Hampshire. She's a hypnotherapist with thirty years experience in education and counseling on the collegiate level and who practices in the private sector.

Based on Dr. Grantly Dick-Read's techniques of natural childbirth, HypnoBirthing is a philosophy and method of confident, calm, and comfortable childbirth. When properly exercised it places the mom in a naturally-induced state of relaxed concentration, a state of mind and body in which she can communicate suggestions to her subconscious mind. It's a powerful and effective form of hypnotherapy. HypnoBirthing helps a mother become deeply relaxed, but at the same time sharply focused and aware during labor and birth. The result is that she experiences little or no discomfort.

HypnoBirthing is an easy-to-learn method of deep relaxation using slow breathing techniques and allowing a laboring woman's body to release its own natural opiates that allow her to experience a medication-free, safe, and gentle birth.

HypnoBirthing prepares the mom physically, mentally, and spiritually for a relaxing and stress-free birth. This program teaches a woman how to go with the natural flow of her own body through labor and birth, allowing her to trust her own birthing abilities and have her baby with little or no pain.

HypnoBirthing teaches that pain is not an automatic part of normal childbirth. It teaches you that your body has its own natural epidural, and shows you how to utilize it. You learn how to achieve relaxation—free of the resistance that fear creates—and how to use your natural birthing instincts for a calm, serene, and comfortable birth.

HypnoBirthing lets you experience a daydream-like effect that will totally relax you. You'll be able to determine the degree to which you'll feel the contractions you're having. You'll be free of the fear and tension that prevents the muscles of your body from functioning as nature intended them to. And all this will allow your body to naturally release endorphins and replace the stress hormones that constrict and cause pain.

And it's really beautiful. When women are properly trained for childbirth and their mind and body are in harmony, nature is free to function in the same well-designed manner. Mothers have a faster and easier birth while retaining energy. They actually achieve a sense of peace and calm that remains throughout the birthing experience.

Although it may sound like it, this isn't a new concept. Hypnotists and MDs have used hypnosis in childbirth for decades, generally for a pain management mindset. And so it is with the HypnoBirthing philosophy—an understanding that birthing isn't supposed to be painful to begin with. These are myths that have created centuries of fear around childbirth in Western cultures. HypnoBirthing offers a very holistic approach to relaxed pregnancy, in utero bonding, and birthing.

> Benefits of HypnoBirthing:
> ◆ Eliminates the fear-tension-pain syndrome before and during birthing
> ◆ Reduces or eliminates the need for analgesics
> ◆ Eliminates fatigue during labor
> ◆ Shortens first stage labor and makes transition a natural part of this stage
> ◆ Brings together mother, baby, and birthing companion in very special pre-, peri-, and post-natal bonding
> ◆ Eliminates hyperventilation caused by shallow breathing methods
> ◆ Returns birthing to a peaceful celebration of life
> ◆ Postnatal recovery is rapid and easier
> ◆ Parents report better bonding with the baby and better-adjusted babies
> ◆ Brings together the whole family
> ◆ Self-hypnosis skills help the stress of parenting and other life aspects

The HypnoBirthing philosophy also includes the knowledge that actual words truly do shape our experience. So different, more gentle, terminology is used—terms that are non-medical and free of negative, painful, and limiting associations. For example, the word "contraction" is a highly-charged word, almost automatically associated with pain. The words "surge," "wave," or "rushes" are used instead. Likewise with the word "pain"; moms say they feel pressure or tightening sensations whenever they hear it. "Water" does not "break," the "membrane releases." The term "medical complication" is replaced with "special circumstances that may need additional attention."

I've read numerous accounts from parents about their HypnoBirthing

> "The most empowering thought to remember about HypnoBirthing is that packages are delivered and pizzas are delivered, but babies are birthed! And the mom is doing the birthing—no one is delivering her a little present." —Marie Mongan

experiences and the same testimonies were repeated over and over: How relaxed they felt... How confident they were when they entered the hospital... How well they were able to interact with their significant others between waves, and how quickly they were able to concentrate when a new rush came. Moms over and over again stated how easy it was to stay focused on the moment and how short their labors were.

The Classes

The training consists of five 2-1/2-hour units taught by an experienced practitioner. The parents learn about hypnosis, self-hypnotic techniques, profound relaxation methods, and how the body is designed to give birth naturally.

UNIT #1: Building a Positive Expectancy

+ Introduction and Philosophy of Gentle Birthing
+ Articles of Birth Affirmation
+ HypnoBirthing Beginnings
+ Rationale for Gentle Birthing/Muscle Comparisons
+ How The Uterus Works
+ How Fear Affects Labor
+ Origin of the Pain Concept
+ Hypnosis and Deep Relaxation
+ Psycho-Physical Relationship
+ HypnoBirthing—Videos #1 and #2

UNIT #2: *Falling in Love with Your Baby/Preparing Mind and Body*

+ HypnoBirthing Stories—Videos #3 and #4
+ Pre-Birth Parenting
+ Relaxation and Breathing
+ Progressive and Instant Relaxation/Deepening Techniques
+ Hypnotic Relaxation and Visualizations
+ Releasing Limiting Thoughts
+ Preparing the Body for Birthing

UNIT #3: *Getting Ready to Welcome Your Baby*

+ Birth Stories—Videos #5 and #6
+ Daddy's Promise
+ Preparing Your Birth Preferences
+ Completing Records and Pre-Admission Registration
+ Assisting in Turning Breech Presentations
+ Looking at an Estimated Due Date
+ Special Circumstances Requiring the Attention of a Care Provider
+ Achieving a Natural Onset of Labor
+ Your Body, Working with You and for You
+ Releasing Negative Emotions, Fears, and Limiting Thoughts

UNIT #4: Overview of Childbirth—A Labor of Love

- ✦ Birth stories—Video #7
- ✦ Prelude to Labor
- ✦ Pre-labor Warm-ups/Practice Labor
- ✦ Onset of Labor—Thinning and Opening Phase
- ✦ Leaving for the Hospital
- ✦ Arriving at the Hospital
- ✦ As Labor Moves Along
- ✦ A Resting or Slowed Labor
- ✦ As Labor Advances—Nearing Completion
- ✦ Birth Rehearsal Imagery

UNIT #5: Birthing—Breathing love, Bringing Life

- ✦ Birth Video—Birth into Being
- ✦ Mother at Completion—Thinning and Opening Phase Ends
- ✦ Birthing Phase Begins—Birth Breathing
- ✦ Birthing Positions
- ✦ Repositioning Baby for Optimal Birthing
- ✦ Birth—The Final Act
- ✦ Family Bonding
- ✦ Post Birth Procedures
- ✦ Clamping/Cutting Cord after Pulsation Stops
- ✦ Birth of Placenta
- ✦ Continued Family Bonding
- ✦ The Fourth Trimester

If you have any other questions, you can visit Mickey's website at *www.HypnoBirthing.com*, or ask your birth professional/doula about classes in your area.

It's clear to me that HypnoBirthing is a fabulous and relaxing way to learn to manage your pregnancy and labor. Using HypnoBirthing seems to be such a serene way to introduce your baby into your life, from prenatal bonding to the actual birthing and beyond.

✦ *REFLEXOLOGY*
AND ACUPRESSURE ✦

Reflexology is an ancient art and science originally practiced by Japanese, Chinese, Indians, and Egyptians over 4,000 years ago. It works by stimulating specific organs of the body through various reflex points on the feet or hands. This encourages the body to help heal itself. Using reflexology on a pregnant mom is safe and extremely relaxing for the mind and body.

Reflexology is excellent for relaxation, lowering blood pressure, stress reduction, increasing energy, improving circulation, and reducing the effects of morning sickness.

Reflexology is a gentle, holistic treatment that introduces harmony and balance to the pregnant woman. By applying pressure to various reflex points it creates a stimulating effect throughout the whole body and causes an energizing effect though the nervous system to the brain.

My own personal experience with reflexology wasn't while I was pregnant but was with my daughter Rayna. Before my daughter had her second heart surgery for repair of a Ventricular Septal Defect (a hole in the lower chamber of her heart), I took her to a reflexologist hoping to find an alternative method to close the hole. When we arrived, and even before the reflexologist took her medical history, he looked into her eyes. By examining their distinguishing marks he correctly diagnosed her condition. He even told me she was starting to exhibit signs of liver failure, which was diagnosed by her medical doctor a couple of weeks later. Unfortunately, the hole in her heart was too large to close using reflexology, but I was so impressed with the art of reflexology that I continued using his services whenever the kids had colds or exhibited flu-like symptoms; it always helped.

With all the changes your body will experience during pregnancy—and let me tell, you there are a lot of them—reflexology is an excellent method of maintaining good health and wellbeing. It can assist in making pregnancy an easier and more "normal" experience for a woman.

Some pregnancies come with several discomforts and stresses. Reflexology can relieve, or lessen, the effects of backache, carpal tunnel syndrome, constipation, fatigue, leg cramps, minor edema, insomnia, and mood swings.

A variation of reflexology, the healing touch of acupressure also reduces tension, increases circulation, and enables the body to let go. Acupressure and reflexology applied to various points of the body can remedy various inconveniences of pregnancy. Acupressure, incorporated with the use of reflexology, will not only help maintain an easier pregnancy but will make your baby's birth less stressful and easier to manage.

Acupressure is also an ancient healing art, developed over 5,000 years ago. The acupressure points are the same points used in acupuncture, but the healing sites are stimulated with finger pressure instead of a needle. Using the power of the hand, acupressure and reflexology are effective in the relief of stress-related ailments, in self-treatment, and in preventive health care. Combined with massage they can relieve tension, increase circulation, and reduce pain.

Listed below are a few ways that acupressure and reflexology can be used to aid in your pregnancy, pain management, and postpartum phase.

Malpresentation of Fetus

Malpresentation of the fetus (especially breech in the 34–36th week of pregnancy) is one of the misfortunes that may lead to a C-section if not corrected. This may be helped with acupressure.

Applying pressure to the outside area of the little toe just below the nail bed can help turn a baby in utero. With mom lying on a flat surface with her feet elevated and head down (Trendelenburg position), use the nail of your index finger and gently scratch the outside portion of the little toe below the nail bed. Stimulate the right foot little toe, then the left foot little toe, each for thirty seconds. Repeat several times, with about a 60-second rest in between. Every third time, rest about 15–20 minutes. This will also help turn a baby that is posterior in labor.

Another method before labor is established when the baby is breech is to tape a grain of uncooked rice on that pressure point.

Pressure to this area during labor can also help the baby move down into position, allowing the labor to progress at a quicker pace.

Induction of Labor

Induction is defined as the initiation of labor before the spontaneous onset for the purpose of accomplishing birth. Artificially inducing labor doesn't always end up with a perfect birth. The British Columbia Reproductive Care Program-Obstetric Guideline warns: "In first-time labor, induction results in twice the risk of cesarean section as compared with spontaneous labor. As well, there's an increased risk of fetal compromise, uterine rupture, and inadvertent delivery of a preterm infant."

Artificially induced labor is more challenging than a spontaneous labor. The use of synthetic oxytocin in combination of prostaglandin gel on the cervix can result in hyper-stimulation of the uterus, causing contractions that are too extreme and intense, far different from the more normal, gradual increase in intensity that accompanies spontaneous labor. Whenever artificial means (medications used for this purpose) are used to stimulate contractions and induce labor, the labor will be intensified and other means of interfering will be necessary to facilitate the birth. With artificial induction, because of this intensity, the baby will need to be continuously monitored, and the likelihood of fetal distress increases. Moms will usually exhibit more pain and might need intervention with more aggressive pain management or epidural—and with each step of intervention this increases the likelihood of having to have a C-section.

IMPORTANT: Sometimes things just get too complicated to be called normal any longer, and aggressive intervention is necessary to save the life of the mom and baby.

I have never seen an induction that didn't lead to lots of other interventions. After Pitocin is administered, the contractions get so severe that a mother usually asks for, and is encouraged to have, an epidural. After the epidural, when the mother is numb from the waist down, the doctor can up the Pitocin dosage to extremely dangerous levels to keep the contractions strong and frequent. The baby will usually start showing signs of distress, so an internal fetal monitor is screwed onto the top of his scalp after the mother's membranes are ruptured. The mother now can't get up, she is constantly monitored, has a Foley catheter in to help her urinate, and will have continuous IVs infusing. The baby will be continually squeezed with strong contractions at a very rapid and intense rate until he is born, most likely exhausted, limp, blue, and needing help to get started. He will nurse poorly and bonding between mother and baby will be compromised.

But there are *other* ways to induce labor if there's a need for it.

If there's a need to start labor or enhance a stalled labor, reflexology and acupressure are less invasive and more gentle to the system. By applying acupressure you can stimulate the pituitary reflex, which helps release the body's own oxytocin, the hormone that induces uterine contractions. At the same time, applying this pressure can be beneficial in giving the stalled uterus a gentle nudge.

To help give the uterus a nudge, and stimulate the release of oxytocin into your system, you can have your birth professional apply pressure with her thumb to the area four finger-widths below the kneecap, and one finger-width outside of the shinbone on both legs for 30–60 seconds. This should be done allowing a couple minutes rest in between to help the mother's body release the much-needed oxytocin. This is effective and less invasive then the use of drugs.

You can also apply pressure to an area four finger-widths above the outer ankle or the tip of the medial malleous with the same effect. This point should be pressed hard with the thumb, coming from behind the ankle. This should be done one leg at a time for about 60 seconds, then after 20–30 minutes apply pressure to the other leg. This isn't a very comfortable place to put pressure, but it does get the contractions started. Applying pressure to these points during labor also keeps the contractions ongoing and steady. <u>CAUTION</u>: This must NEVER be done during your pregnancy, as it can cause an early labor.

Pain Management

Here's great news: Because they're a form of reflexology, foot and hand massages really do help when it comes to managing discomfort during labor. So go for it, ladies; you've been validated.

There are also a couple of acupressure points to try. On the back of the ankle, between the inner protrusion of the anklebone and the Achilles tendon, is an area that, when stimulated during labor, can help to relieve labor and backaches. Pressing this area between your thumb and forefinger for 60 seconds at a time, with rest in between, will help relieve discomfort.

Another one that works well with all kinds of discomfort is called the Hoku point, which lies in the webbing between the thumb and index finger. Place your thumb (of the opposite hand, of course) on the top of the web on the back of the hand and squeeze it with your index finger underneath for 30–60 seconds, rest a few minutes, and repeat. This works well with headaches too.

Postpartum

The woman's body faces a lot of challenges when recovering from labor and birthing. The same acupressure points used in releasing oxytocin into the system (the acupressure points below the knee) are also very helpful in strengthening and toning the muscles. They help digestion, can relieve fatigue, and may even stop excessive sweating that can sometimes occur after childbirth.

At the back of the book there is some reading material listed that will give you more information about reflexology and acupressure. Also, in the acknowledgements section, you may find a caregiver in your area that specializes in reflexology.

✦ *YOGA* ✦

A lot of the material I received on yoga in relationship to pregnancy and birthing came from a very experienced yoga instructor, Laura Sevika Douglass, in Watertown, Maine. Below is some of the material she sent me.

More and more caregivers are recommending yoga to their moms— and with good reason… I've seen it work wonders in helping moms to totally relax and focus exclusively on their births. Sometimes couples achieve such complete harmony I can just stand back and marvel at how well they are handling their birth.

Yoga teaches you how to focus on what you're feeling and how to let go and concentrate on what your body is going through. It allows you to relax and accept the process that's taking place, reduces your discomfort, and makes it easier for you to cope with all the changes your body is going through.

With labor, a woman needs to prepare herself for a long journey. She needs supportive people around her, and she needs the knowledge that will make it a less fearful and a more spiritual journey. Yoga connects her with her spiritual side and helps guide her through the sensations she is experiencing with her contractions, avoiding that first instinct to tense-up that can cause her discomfort. The very best way to cope with labor is to accept whatever happens to you and then surrender to it voluntarily. In other words, the art of getting through labor is to relax and trust your body.

> When starting any exercise or activity you have never done before, it's best to wait until after your first trimester. This allows your body to adjust to being pregnant before you introduce other new things.

Taking prenatal yoga classes will help prepare you for pregnancy and childbirth. One form of yoga that's ideal is called Integral Yoga Hatha. It's a combination of postures, Kegel exercises, using sound to relieve tension, breathing practices, deep relaxation, and meditation. But there are many other forms of yoga that practice similar techniques. Ask your caregiver which she uses, or supports, and what classes she recommends.

Breathing

It's almost impossible to remember all the different stages, levels, and kinds of breathing in labor. Yoga teaches you to allow your instincts to take over, and to bring awareness to your breathing. This lets you spontaneously have the power to breathe during your labor without imposing any restrictions.

Inhaling should be as deep as comfortably possible. By taking deep breaths and exhaling completely you provide you and your baby with seven times more oxygen then you would with shallow breathing, giving both of you a great deal of energy. Deep breaths soothe and quiet the entire nervous system. Between contractions, deep breathing helps to calm; during contractions, it helps to relieve fear and panic.

Exhaling is related to surrendering yourself and your energy to the universe and cosmic energy. It helps ease tension and the instinct to hold your breath during a strong contraction. As contractions become stronger many women find it helpful to incorporate deep sounds into their exhaling. In your prenatal yoga classes you will learn about sounds and breathing; it's an excellent idea to practice this prior to labor.

Mantras

A mantra is a repetition of words or phases that have a particular meaning for an individual. In yoga, they serve as "lifeboats" during stressful times. Come up with your own mantra for your baby's birth and teach it to your caregiver and birth attendants. It can come in very handy if you begin feeling any doubts or fears about your labor.

But more than just a lifeboat for you, your mantra will be among the first sounds your baby will hear. Both of you will be going through an intense and amazing experience, and a mantra, chanted with emotion, can help quell the fears of your new child the same way it does for you, and help set the tone of your baby's life.

Postnatal

Fifteen minutes a day of Integral Yoga Hatha will help the new mother regain her strength and flexibility. The postures help revive her vitality and energy, and the meditation and breathing practices help her to stay calm, focused, and open through the many changes of motherhood.

There are also yoga exercises that are wonderful for the baby. They love being touched, and this kind of yoga focuses on gentle massages and movements of their wrists, ankles, arms, and legs. The exercises are safe for all infants and, in some cases, have even helped with constipation.

Babies are fully conscious beings and are very expressive and communicative. In the first few years of life they're in touch with their divine or spiritual energy. During this time new mothers should learn to open themselves to their baby's love, wisdom, and guidance.

Summary

Yoga, reflexology, acupressure, and HypnoBirthing are all aids that are readily available to us as new mothers. We now have easy access to different styles of pregnancy and labor management, and we have some wonderful teachers to show us all the techniques. Allowing the Old World ways into our birthing process helps ground us. It gently brings us back to nature and the natural way of bringing our children into the world. We should embrace every opportunity to explore all our options.

6

Vaginal Birth After Cesarean

◆

At the Risk of Repeating Myself —
"Hey! Who's Having
This Baby Anyway?"

"If you think you can, you can. And if you think you can't, you're right."
  —Mary Kay Ash

I've included this chapter because there's a growing concern that cesarean births are increasing at an alarming rate. In the 1970s the cesarean rate was 5% of births in the United States. In 2003 the Center for Disease Control stated it was up to 27.6%—that's more then one in four women birthing their children by cesarean. This increase was coming from an era when the standard of thinking was, "Once a cesarean, always a cesarean." This is no longer the case. Yes, if it was anatomically necessary, chances are that subsequent births will also have to be by cesarean. But if the reason was maternal or because of extended labor, malpresentation, fetal distress, or just a doctor in a hurry, the chances are excellent that the next baby can be born vaginally. So why the alarming increase?

It's the lack of real support, sincere encouragement, and an honest opportunity that prevents women from seeking vaginal births after C-sections. As a result, 40% of birthing women with a prior cesarean don't attempt a vaginal birth in their next pregnancy.

Women deserve and need to be told they can birth their babies vaginally, naturally, and joyfully.

This chapter includes some information from the International Cesarean Awareness Network, Inc. (ICAN), a wonderful non-profit organization founded by Esther Booth Zorn in 1982. ICAN has been doing a great job of educating moms and helping them increase their chances of avoiding unnecessary cesareans and having a vaginal births. This organization also supports Vaginal Births After Cesareans (VBAC). I want to thank them for giving me permission to use some of the following information.

The ICAN of VBAC
and the 'I Can't' of ACOG

In a newsletter, ICAN stated the following:

> The CDC (Center for Disease Control) said 27.6 percent of U.S. women birthed their babies via cesarean in 2002, the highest ever reported in the United States. This marked a seven-percent increase over 2001. According to the World Health Organization (WHO), cesarean rates above 15 percent represent a danger to women and babies. ICAN attributes the U.S. cesarean increase to the wide availability of elective cesareans and the elimination of vaginal birth after cesarean (VBAC) options at some hospitals due to changes in American College of Obstetricians and Gynecologists (ACOG)* guidelines.

In July 1999, ACOG issued an updated practice bulletin on VBAC, replacing their previous recommendations of October 1998. The previous bulletin called for a surgeon to be "readily available" when a woman with a prior cesarean was in labor. This meant that if a woman with a previous cesarean was in labor and wanted to have her baby vaginally a surgical team had to be available within 30 minutes to perform a C-section if there were any problems. The 1999 guidelines changed this to recommend a "physician immediately available throughout active labor capable of monitoring labor and performing an immediate cesarean." This means that there has to be a surgical team with an operating room set up and ready during the woman's whole laboring process. But surgical teams are not willing to hang out in the hospital waiting for a woman to birth her baby, so most hospitals are refusing to offer VBAC services. Some hospitals are giving their laboring moms time limits— if they birth their baby before the surgical team leaves the hospital they can have their baby vaginally. The practice bulletin also states that a contraindication to VBAC would be "inability to perform emergency cesarean birth because of unavailable surgeon, anesthesia, sufficient staff, or facility."

"Whether one agrees or disagrees with the new ACOG guidelines it is important to remember that ACOG is not a college in the sense of an institution of higher learning, nor is it a scientific body, it is a professional organization that in reality is one kind of trade union. Like every trade union, ACOG has two goals: promote the interests of its members, and promote a better product (in this case, the wellbeing of women). But if there is conflict between these two goals the interests of obstetricians come first."

—Critique of ACOG Practice Bulletin # 5, July 1999, "Vaginal birth after previous cesarean section" by Marsden Wagner, MD, MSPH

This is what occurred and continues to occur in one hospital I am familiar with. Although a recipient of the Coalition for Improving Maternity Services (CIMS) certificate, they won't let a VBAC mother labor without a full surgical staff in the hospital at the time. Anesthesiologists and obstetricians balk at having to be in-house during the night, so the physicians are discouraging previous cesarean women from laboring and birthing vaginally. But with the pressure from the mothers, maternity staff, and unit nurse managers, things are slowly coming around. This may have a happy ending for previous cesarean moms.

Physicians and hospitals feel that failure to adhere to the ACOG guidelines could leave them open to malpractice suits in the unlikely event of a uterine rupture, causing harm to the mother or baby. Statistically, a VBAC is relatively risk-free for both mother and infant. Henci Goer's research of studies on VBACs show that there were just 46 ruptures in 15,154 labors. This works out to a risk of only one-third of one percent (0.3%). And Dr. Mark Landon writes that the overall risk for a serious newborn complication is only approximately 1 in 2,000 trials of labor (.05%).

When we compare this to some of the other risks that a laboring mom routinely faces, the over-cautious reaction to a 0.3% chance of rupture looks ridiculous. The research I have found shows the following:

+ Cord prolapse (when the umbilical cord slips through the cervix before the baby) occurs in 1 out of 37 births (2.7%), or nearly ten times more likely than that of rupture.

+ The recurrence rate for women who have had a placenta previa (when the placenta blocks the birth canal) is 4 to 8%.

+ You are 6 times more likely to have a doctor who is an impostor than you are to suffer a rupture (2% of doctors [1 in 50] are phonies).

+ This is not a risk but fun to know: the chances of having twins are 3-1/2 times greater (odds of twins: 1 in 90).

Given these statistics, I'm surprised ACOG isn't insisting that *every* birth should have a surgical team available!

But as I said before, most of the time the 0.3% risk excuse is only what providers tell you, and not the real reason for denying you a VBAC. Surgical

Potential Problems Associated
With Cesarean Births

✦ Injury to maternal bladder
   or bowel

✦ Extension of uterine incision
   into uterine arteries, cervix,
   or vagina

✦ Uterine atony (lack of normal
   muscle tone)

✦ Dense adhesions from
   previous surgery

✦ Hemorrhage from placental
   implantation site

✦ Uterine rupture

✦ Endomyometritis

✦ Wound infection
   or hematoma

Potential Complications

✦ Patient's age

✦ Number of previous
   pregnancies

✦ Medical problems
   during pregnancy

✦ Clinical reason(s) for
   cesarean birth

✦ Physician's role in surgery;
   i.e. primary surgeon, first or
   second assistant

✦ Type of skin incision and type
   of uterine incision

✦ Infant Apgar score
   and weight

✦ Occurrence of
   postoperative infection

✦ Surgical complications

teams simply don't want the inconvenience of having to be available after hours. It's no coincidence that the vast majority of "emergency" C-sections happen during the 40 hours between 9 to 5 on weekdays and not during the other 128 hours of the week.

And if you question his order for a cesarean, the provider usually replies with a statement like, "Do you want to take the chance of having a dead baby?" or, "You're putting your baby in danger if you try to birth vaginally." So you need to remember what his definition of "chance" and "danger" is—0.3%. *You have a 99.7% chance of not having a ruptured uterus if you birth your baby vaginally after a previous cesarean.*

But if you did end up having the cesarean, you would naturally assume that the 0.3% risk would disappear and you'd be risk-free. Well you couldn't be more wrong. You also need to know that by insisting on a cesarean, your provider is actually exposing you to a much higher risk.

For example, the National Institute of Health (NIH) states that maternal morbidity (illness following the procedure) is five to ten times *higher* for cesarean than vaginal birth. Morbidity rates include, but are not limited to, operative injuries, operative and post-operative hemorrhage, pulmonary emboli (blood clot in the lung), venous thrombosis (sluggish blood flow), anesthesia complications, and infection. There have been rates as high as 50% morbidity associated with cesareans.

The NIH also states that mortality (death) rates are four times higher in cesarean births than in vaginal birth, and that a repeat cesarean carries twice the risk of maternal mortality than VBAC does.

Other risks for mom include hysterectomy, surgical mistakes, re-hospitalization, and dangerous placental abnormalities in future pregnancies.

Repeat cesareans are linked to a host of risks for baby as well: low birth weight, prematurity, respiratory problems, and lacerations. ICAN believes a repeat

2002 CESAREAN RATES (percentage) BY STATE (all races)

State	Rate	State	Rate
United States	26.1	Nebraska	26.7
Alabama	28.7	Nevada	25.7
Alaska	19.4	New Hampshire	24.1
Arizona	21.3	New Jersey	30.9
Arkansas	29.1	New Mexico	19.1
California	26.8	New York	27.2
Colorado	21.1	North Carolina	26.3
Connecticut	26.1	North Dakota	23.1
Delaware	27.3	Ohio	23.4
District of Columbia	26.6	Oklahoma	28.1
Florida	28.5	Oregon	23.4
Georgia	25.9	Pennsylvania	24.9
Hawaii	21.4	Rhode Island	26.0
Idaho	19.7	South Carolina	28.6
Illinois	23.9	South Dakota	24.6
Indiana	24.9	Tennessee	27.5
Iowa	24.8	Texas	27.9
Kansas	24.8	Utah	19.1
Kentucky	27.8	Vermont	21.1
Louisiana	30.4	Virginia	26.8
Maine	25.7	Washington	24.0
Maryland	27.5	West Virginia	29.3
Massachusetts	28.0	Wisconsin	20.6
Michigan	24.9	Wyoming	21.1
Minnesota	22.2	Puerto Rico	44.7
Mississippi	31.1	Virgin Islands	22.1
Missouri	25.7	Guam	20.4 (2)
Montana	23.0		

Source: National Vital Statistics Reports Vol. 51, Number 11, Table 7

cesarean should never be considered routine. It is major abdominal surgery with many risks.

The plain fact is that all physicians take an oath to "do no harm"—which means choosing a path of least risk to patients. Yet unnecessary elective cesareans *increase* risks to birthing women. It seems plainly unethical and inappropriate for obstetricians to perform unnecessary surgery on a healthy woman with a normal pregnancy—and this includes a repeat cesarean.

It's high time that we ask ourselves what kind of a provider would ignore his oath and subject a laboring woman to higher risks just for his personal convenience and the convenience of his colleagues.

Preparing for a VBAC

Okay, you know the facts, you've read the reasoning, and now you need to do your homework to prepare yourself for a VBAC.

To begin your quest to have a vaginal birth after you had your last baby by cesarean, you need to begin planning at the start of your pregnancy. You will need to create a habit of good nutrition and ongoing moderate exercise. Start at the library, a bookstore, or Amazon.com to borrow or buy and read the prenatal and pregnancy books I've listed in the back—they have some great guidelines on nutrition for pregnant moms. You might want to consider keeping a daily nutritional journal or checklist to ensure you are getting the essential nutrients and vitamins you need. Engage in some form of daily exercise, such as swimming, walking, yoga, or a prenatal fitness class—whatever feels good and whatever encourages you to exercise every day. Of course, readers are strongly cautioned to consult with a health care professional before beginning any exercise regime.

Become informed. Register with VBAC. They have a website at www.vbac.com that is full of useful information. Classes are a must for success, and it's also a good idea to attend VBAC support meetings. Join other local and national organizations. Through these gatherings you'll meet with other parents that are striving for an alternative to their last cesarean—they may even have some wonderful connections to doulas, providers, and birth attendants that can help you.

Also please read *The VBAC Companion* by Diana Korte and *The VBAC Experience* by Lynn Baptisti Richards, a collection of very helpful VBAC stories.

Find a provider that will give you a chance to have a trial labor with liberal guidelines. Know your statistics and write down researched information to show to your provider; this will show him or her that you are well educated and know what you want.

Women have commonly been denied trials of labor if their first cesarean section was performed for failure to progress (FTP) or cephalopelvic disproportion (CPD), the most common indications for primary cesarean as cited in a 1987 study published in the American Journal of Public Health. Of these women, 65 percent—almost two-thirds—went on to have normal births. —ICAN Clarion, September 1997.

Research shows that approximately 80 percent of women who have given birth by cesarean will be able to go on to give birth vaginally. (Some studies even show success rates of over 90 percent!) Over 75 percent of the birthing women who were originally diagnosed with CPD or FTP were successful in their attempts to have a VBAC with their subsequent birth. One third of these women gave birth to a larger baby than their first.

This was from a featured article on VBAC from iVillage.

It is possible to have your baby vaginally after a cesarean—research and statistics prove this. I could list a lot more articles, but I'm going to let you jump onto the Internet to find them for yourself. Just remember that to be successful with a vaginal birth after a cesarean, there is still more planning you'll have to do.

First, find the right help. When hiring a doctor, be sure he is supportive of what your wishes are and shows encouragement. Ask if he believes in VBACs and if he has a VBAC success rate of over 75 percent and a cesarean rate that is lower then the community average, which is around 25 percent. Find a hospital and doctor that ALREADY provide the options you want. Make sure they have a 24-hour surgery team in case you develop problems. You might want to consider hiring a midwife as your primary caregiver; midwives have a very low rate of cesarean births. I really encourage you to talk with other parents who have had a successful VBAC and ask who their doctor was and which hospital they chose. If you are unsure about anything, get a second opinion and trust your inner strength and knowledge. Don't fall into believing the fear tactics that some providers offer—make them show you statistics and proof.

Below are helpful tips and a checklist from ICAN. You can also find this on their website and print it out to have with you when you go interviewing.

How to Choose
a Doctor or Midwife
Checklists and Tips for Interviewing

How much do we put our bodies, our health, and ourselves into the hands of doctors we hardly know? How will they handle a certain situation? How much medical intervention do they think we need? How much is too much? Do you know her preferences? Does she know yours? Take the time to ask questions and get the answers. Know and listen to your body. Make decisions about your birth instead of leaving it to the doctor's discretion. Do you trust your doctor? Take the time to find a doctor that respects and honors your opinions.

Where Does a Doctor Stand?

To find out where a doctor stands on issues important to you, pick two, and ask the questions at your next visit. Have them written down and have a pen to write down the answers. You should never be made to feel like the questions you ask are unimportant or that you are rushed. You are finding out about your care.

Making An Appointment With a New Doctor

Call and tell the receptionist you are looking for a new doctor and just want to talk to the doctor or midwife. Tell them again when you go to the office.

Talking to the Doctor or Midwife

Emphasize you don't want or need an exam; you're simply going to talk. Have a list of questions ready. Be clear about your concerns and requests. Tailor your questions to the information you need from your doctor or midwife. What are your issues? Do you want support for a VBAC? Do you want your birth to be a natural birth? It's always a good idea to know who the backup doctors are and what their policies are. If you're pregnant, find out if your doctor/midwife has a vacation scheduled near your due date.

Ten Interview Questions for a Doctor or Certified Nurse Midwife

1. Approximately how many VBACs have you attended?

2. Of those patients in your practice who wanted VBACs, how many were successful?

3. What do you think my chances are of VBAC success, given my childbirth history?

4. What is your cesarean rate?

5. How do you usually manage a postdate pregnancy or a suspected cephalopelvic disproportion?

6. What's a reasonable length of time for a VBAC labor if I'm healthy and my baby appears to be healthy?

7. What percentage of your patient's babies do you catch yourself?

8. How many people can I have with me during the labor and birth?

9. What is your usual recommendation for IVs, Pitocin, prostaglandin gel, amniotomy, epidurals, confinement to bed, EFM (and so on)?

10. How close together are your appointments?

The above questions were taken from Diana Korte's book *The VBAC Companion: The Expectant Mother's Guide to Vaginal Birth After Cesarean* (Harvard Common Press, 1998), a must-have book for moms considering that option.

More Questions for Obstetricians

✦ How often do women in your care give birth without medication? How many with minimal medication? In what percentage of your patients do you induce labor?

✦ What is your episiotomy rate? How many mothers birth over an intact perineum? What is your percentage of forceps birth or vacuum extraction?

✦ How long have you been in practice? What are your credentials?

✦ At what hospitals do you have privileges?

✦ Is your practice group or solo? If group, do all the doctors share the same philosophy and practices?

✦ What prenatal tests/procedures do you require or recommend?

✦ How do you feel about labor support persons other than my partner?

✦ How many of your patients give birth in a squatting, standing, hands and knees, or side-lying position?

✦ Do you have any vacations planned near my due date?

✦ What book(s) would you recommend that I read?

✦ What would you suggest if my baby were breech?

✦ Are you planning to be at the hospital with me as I labor?

✦ On a first-time mom, how many hours do you give her to labor before you intervene?

✦ Do you break waters just to speed up labor when you come to check a mom during labor?

✦ Do you routinely use Pitocin to increase contractions if labor is slower then you would expect?

Thank you, ICAN, for permission to use this material.

When attempting a VBAC it's especially important that you hire a doula, labor assistant, or other trained and qualified support person. It's worth every penny to hire someone who believes that birth is a natural function and to be there for you with support and care. This helper should be present with you during your labor at home, your birth in the hospital, and through your post-partum phase. They'll also take the pressure off dad and family members so the whole family can be supportive.

Have a Birth Plan

Prior to your baby's birth, I strongly encourage you to write a birth plan (see the Birth Plan section, Chapter 9, in this book). Discuss EVERYTHING that is important to you with your care provider, and then follow it up by putting it all in writing. Make extra copies to put in your chart and be sure you and your doula each have one to bring to the hospital. It's wise to know your hospital's VBAC policies beforehand and to discuss these policies in depth when you negotiate your wishes with your doctor and the nurse manager where you will have your baby. And be sure your provider signs the hospital's copy.

What to consider when writing your birth plan:

+ Establish a safe and supportive birth environment to encourage labor. State who you want at your birth and how you want the room to look (dim lights, music, no students at your birth, etc.).

+ Try a variety of positions during labor and pushing. Instead of lying down, try standing or walking. Try the birth ball. Squatting to push can be most effective. Try walking in the halls. Heck, you might even try "dancing" with your partner.

+ Continue your calorie and fluid intake. Labor is work and takes energy. Far from eliminating the risk of aspiration with general anesthesia, total fasting may increase the risk of raising acidity in the stomach. You want your nutrition to be received orally and not through an IV.

✦ Avoid unnecessary medical intervention whenever possible. Continuous electronic fetal monitoring may restrict your movement. Ask for noninvasive options. Ask what will be done with the results.

✦ Artificial induction should be avoided. Medical induction is linked to high rupture rates and many interventions.

✦ Ask for additional time to try non-medical methods to stimulate labor if it is not progressing. These include change of position, walking, nipple stimulation, aromatherapy, acupressure, and reflexology. Every labor is different. Unless you dilated to 5 or 6 centimeters during a previous birth and before your cesarean, consider this one as your first. If your labor was interrupted before you reached 5 cm then your body had not actually experienced a true labor or birth so it would be treating this labor as your first.

✦ Avoid epidurals. They decrease your chance for a vaginal birth. Epidurals interfere with the baby getting optimally aligned and will reduce your ability to push effectively. It has also been known to slow or stop labor. Try natural pain relief measures such as hot/cold compresses, a bath or shower, Tenns units, massage, relaxation, guided imagery, HypnoBirthing techniques, yoga, and the birth ball. If you start to feel you'll need an epidural, give yourself a few more contractions, or request that you be checked one more time. You may be moving quickly into transition without realizing it.

What it all comes down to is getting the support you need for your next birth after a cesarean. You may have a fear that your body might "fail" again. During labor you'll reach the point when your previous birth was arrested, and pushing past this point requires a great deal of trust in the birth process and encouragement from those around you.

Trusting your body's ability to give birth is not as simple as it may seem. Knowing that you have a 75 percent chance of giving birth vaginally can be overshadowed if your birth experience is 100% cesarean. You know no other outcome, and your previous experience will lead your mind down the more familiar path.

So above all, believe in yourself and the birth process. Keep encouraging yourself, saying you *are* capable of birthing your baby vaginally. Get in touch with the inner you—your resources and abilities—and focus on the positive aspects of your pregnancy. Continue working on leftover negative emotions (guilt, disappointment, anger) from your previous cesarean births. Learn to trust, cooperate with, and listen to your body and baby. Listen for your own unique labor pattern. And in general, just feel good about yourself!

Following the ideas at the beginning of this chapter will help prepare you. Nutrition, exercise, seeking prenatal classes and support, choosing a doctor and hospital with high VBAC rates, and writing a birth plan are all beginnings of a vaginal birth. But mainly, having someone there to support you and keep you on track throughout your labor and birth will help bring about the best possible outcome. And remember, success shouldn't be measured by how you had your baby—whether vaginally or by cesarean. Success is measured by birthing a healthy baby to a healthy mom—no matter how it came into the world.

Tips on Post-Cesarean Healing

With the help of an article from ICAN, here some tips to healing after your cesarean.

Make no mistake about it, cesarean birth is major abdominal surgery. New mothers need (and deserve) to have extra support during this special time of birth and healing. Women who have experienced either a planned or unplanned cesarean react to the surgery in very individual ways—some heal very quickly while others report that recovery took several weeks or months. Avoid putting time limits on yourself and let your body heal in its own good time.

Emotionally, women's feelings about their cesareans vary from acceptance to disappointment to devastation. Some need as much emotional support as physical support for a healthy recovery and growth into the new role of motherhood.

Above all, hiring a postpartum doula during this time of physical and emotional recovery is very important for the mother and her family.

To Relieve Pain and Assist Physical Healing:

At the hospital: Ask for physical assistance when you need to turn or pick up your baby, and always keep the nurse call-button within easy reach. It's also nice to have a family member spend the night with you the first night to jump up and help you when you need it.

For the first couple of days, schedule your pain medication every 2–3 hours to keep the discomfort under control. After that, take it as needed. Avoid codeine, which causes constipation. (T3—Tylenol 3—has codeine in it.) I find that Vicodin is the most tolerated and effective pain medication.

If possible, obtain a private room so that a family member can remain with you. You can usually order one when you pre-register at the hospital, but most hospitals now are doing rooming-in care and only have one room per mother.

Use pillows to support your abdomen when turning, standing, coughing, and when feeding your baby. Bring a small couch pillow with you to the hospital for tummy support when you're up.

Rest as much as possible and limit visitors. Sleep when baby sleeps. It's okay to have the nurses put a "Do Not Disturb" sign on your door during the day when you're napping. Have the ward clerk in the hospital put a hold on all your phone calls for at least two hours in the afternoon for a good nap.

Rock in a rocking chair as soon as possible after surgery to speed up recovery and reduce gas.

Take short walks. Each time you stand up and stretch it helps un-cramp stomach muscles and makes the next time you're up easier.

Eat nutritious food and drink plenty of fluids. Avoid cold and carbonated beverages because they create gas and could make you very uncomfortable. Also, stay away from straws—they encourage the intake of air and cause gas.

The surgery will slow down your digestive tract. To help with constipation, try a stool softener, NOT a laxative. Hospitals usually give you a mild stool softener at night before you go to bed. If not, ask them to have one ordered for you.

Check the incision frequently for signs of infection. Report to your doctor any symptoms of increased pain, swelling, redness, or discharge. The nurse will keep track of any change in your fever that could indicate an infection.

At Home: Have several diapering stations located around the house so you can change your baby easily. Consider having a diaper service; the cost is about the same as disposable diapers, and it's friendlier to the environment and nicer on your baby's bottom.

Let others do household chores like cooking, cleaning, and laundry. When friends come, it's okay to give them something to do while they're visiting. If you feel uncomfortable asking for help, keep a list of things needing to be done and ask your visitors to choose something from the list they would be willing to do.

Remember not to lift anything heavier than your baby for the first two weeks.

Stay in your pajamas, so people remember that you're recovering from birth and surgery.

On the other hand, sometimes taking a shower and getting dressed really does wonders psychologically. Even in the hospital, it can help to put on your own clothes.

Keep the baby near you at night so you do not have to get up. A helpful idea is for your partner to change the baby at night and hand him to you to nurse. If your baby is bottle-fed, the night feeding can be a very special time for your partner and baby to get to know each other, not to mention allowing you a couple extra hours of sleep.

Have a basket that you can carry around easily with nutritious snacks, fingernail clippers, lotion, a book, and other little necessities in it.

Eat well and drink water freely. Keep a pitcher of water or juice near you. Drink a full glass of water or juice every time you nurse or feed your baby.

If you have other children, get help in caring for them from family and friends. A friend taking your little tike to the park while you and the new baby sleep will make for a nice afternoon.

Increase activity gradually. Sometimes when you feel good it is easy to overdo things and end up experiencing a relapse later on. Take care of yourself and, at least for the first week, get plenty of bed rest.

And above all, hire a postpartum doula to do all your chores, help with breastfeeding, and help take care of you and your needs.

To Promote Emotional Healing:

Keep your baby near you as much as possible and get to know him.

Breastfeed your baby to promote bonding and release beneficial mothering hormones.

Share your feelings with others and your partner, and talk about your experience as much as you feel necessary—especially if it was not a planned cesarean.

It is normal to experience a wide range of emotions, including relief, happiness, sadness, anger, and feelings of loss and failure.

Write your baby's birth story. This is one thing that I share with my children at every birthday is their birth story. One year I decided that they were too old to do this, but they called me up and asked for it.

Write letters to the hospital and your doctor, explaining what you did and didn't like about your birth. You can mail them or not, as you choose, but it is beneficial to write your thoughts down either way.

Seek support from available resources including breastfeeding, parental, and cesarean support groups.

Read books on natural childbirth, cesarean birth, and VBAC. There are many reasons why a birth may have ended in a cesarean section. If you plan to have any more children, it is important for you to know that it is very likely you can have a vaginal birth next time. When you're ready to learn about VBAC, ICAN can help you find the information and support you need.

And remember, no matter how you have your baby, vaginally or by C-section, your main goal is to have a healthy baby and a good outcome.

Research and reading will help you succeed in a VBAC. Some books that may help you are listed below.

- ✦ Mancy Cohen, Lois J. Estner, *Silent Knife: Cesarean Prevention and Vaginal Birth after Cesarean,* Bergin and Garvey, 1983
- ✦ Carl Jones, *Expectant Parent's Guide to Preventing a Cesarean Section,* Greenwood Pub Group, 1991
- ✦ Diana Korte, *The VBAC Companion* and *A Good Birth, A Safe Birth: Choosing and Having the Childbirth Experience You Want,* Harvard Common Press, 1992
- ✦ Karis Crawford, Johanne C. Walters, *Natural Childbirth After Cesarean,* Blackwell Science Inc, 1996
- ✦ Claudia Panuthos, *Rebounding From Childbirth* and *Ended Beginnings,* Bergin and Garvey, 1994

VBAC

This worksheet isn't for everyone, just the moms with the desire to have a vaginal birth after they had a cesarean. Incorporate these thoughts into your basic birth plan—there's a lot of work involved in accomplishing a VBAC, not only physically, but in researching and finding a physician and facility that will give you the opportunity. So let's start with finding who can help and where you will be able to do this.

The ideal provider you'll need for a VBAC:

✦ will commit to give you all the time you need to have your baby vaginally;

✦ will be available if you go into labor, even if he's not on call;

✦ will be willing to stay in the hospital with you while you're laboring;

✦ will not put a time limit on your labor;

✦ will not augment your labor with Pitocin or other drugs; and

✦ will openly support your desire to birth your baby vaginally.

As you find physicians that meet most or all of these requirements, list them below.

Name _____

Telephone _____

Office Address _____

_____

Hospital _____

Name _____

Telephone _____

Office Address _____

_____

Hospital _____

Name _____

Telephone _____

Office Address _____

_____

Hospital _____

Name _____

Telephone _____

Office Address _____

_____

Hospital _____

Next you'll need to find a clinic or hospital that will support your VBAC wishes. If your regular hospital won't support VBAC, you'll need to find a birthing clinic or smaller community hospital that will have a surgical staff available 24/7 in case you need a cesarean, and will support your desire to deliver your baby vaginally.

Institution _____

Telephone _____

Address _____

_____

Institution _____

Telephone _____

Address _____

_____

Institution _____

Telephone _____

Address _____

_____

Institution _____

Telephone _____

Address _____

_____

Questions for the Provider

		Yes	No
1.	How many VBACs have you done? _____		
2.	How many of them have birthed vaginally during the night? _____		
3.	Do you work where there is a surgical team available all night?	❏	❏
4.	Do you ever augment laboring VBAC moms with medical interventions?	❏	❏
5.	Do you stay in the hospital while a VBAC mom is laboring?	❏	❏
6.	How long do you allow a VBAC mom to labor? _____		

	Yes	No

7. Why would you choose to perform a cesarean
    on a VBAC mom? _____

8. What is your VBAC rate? _____

9. After reading my medical record, how successful
    do you think I'll be with a vaginal birth? _____

10. What are your policies regarding Pitocin, prostaglandin
    gel (used to ripen the cervix for dilation), epidurals,
    confinement to bed, external fetal monitoring, etc?

    _____

    _____

11. Do the other doctors in your group share your views
    about VBAC?   ❏   ❏

Questions for Yourself

Although we've gone over them before, these points
are a must for a successful VBAC.

	Yes	No

1. Prenatally, I'll exercise and be very aware
    of my nutritional needs.   ❏   ❏

2. I'll have a birth plan ready for my doctor to sign
    prior to labor.   ❏   ❏

3. I will establish a good, safe environment for my baby's
    birth and will have these people with me who support
    my desires:

    _____

    _____

    _____

    _____

	Yes	No

4. I will try different positions to help my labor:

Birth Ball ❑ ❑

Walking ❑ ❑

Squatting ❑ ❑

Tub ❑ ❑

Shower ❑ ❑

Lying on my side ❑ ❑

5. I will bring the following for nourishment:

_____

_____

6. During early labor I want the fetal monitor on for no longer than _____ minutes every hour (you'll need to be up and moving around).

7. Barring emergencies, I'll refuse augmentation or induction no matter how often they're offered. ❑ ❑

If confronted with this, I'll try instead:

Reflexology ❑ ❑

Acupressure ❑ ❑

Nipple stimulation ❑ ❑

Aromatherapy ❑ ❑

8. Before I use any pain medication I first want my cervix checked to see how far I've dilated. ❑ ❑

9. I do not want any pain medications before 5 cm. ❑ ❑

10. I don't want a time limit placed on my labor. ❑ ❑

Other questions I'll ask of myself and my physician and institution:

_____

_____

_____

_____

_____

_____

It's important to remember that because of your prior cesarean, you won't have the choice of refusing a heplock (IV access). But make sure the staff is aware that they may not start any medications or IV fluids without your permission.

Please keep in mind that, above everything else, to have a successful VBAC you must have a committed support team—your partner, friends, birthing professional, physician, and institution—all believing in you and your wishes.

7
Homebirth

◆

More Comfortable Than a Hospital,
Cleaner Than a Rice Patty.

"Life is a matter of preparation meeting opportunity."
—Oprah Winfrey

*T*aking total control of your pregnancy and having your baby at home—your way—is the most extraordinary birthing option of all. Contrary to popular belief, this option isn't as radical as you may think. *A full 95 percent of the people alive in the world today were born at home.*

With proper prenatal care, a carefully chosen midwife, a birth professional or doctor who will attend you at home, and a backup plan in case of an emergency, you can have a successful and safe homebirth, if it's what you really want. Settling on this option isn't an irresponsible choice, it's legal, very much supported and, truth be told, a completely responsible decision when moms and their partners truly apply themselves to doing the right things to prepare. But if homebirth is your choice, you must educate yourself, do your research, hire responsible practitioners who support your wishes, and maintain a healthy pregnancy.

Birthing your baby at home is a beautiful experience packed with love and support from people who are there to help you. Being in familiar surroundings makes birth flow so much better. You'll have access to your favorite quiet retreats, your private garden to stroll in, and the bathtub you love so much. It's comforting to know you won't have to pack up to come home after you have your baby—you're already where you should be when your amazing little package comes into the world.

Homebirth by the Numbers

Statistics have proven that, compared with hospital births, homebirths are safer for both the mother and baby. I am not aware of any statistics showing that hospital birth ensures a better outcome for you or your baby. In fact, the opposite is true. Having a baby in the hospital has been shown to be more dangerous and life threatening than having a baby at home with professional help.

Again, because of its importance, I want to remind you of one of the most comprehensive studies to date that compares hospital birth outcomes to homebirth outcomes was conducted by Dr. Lewis Mehl and associates in 1976.[*1] The study compared 1,046 homebirths with 1,046 hospital births of equivalent populations in the United States. For each homebirth patient, a hospital-birth patient was matched for age, length of gestation, parity (number of pregnancies), risk factor score, education and socioeconomic status, race, presentation of the baby, and individual major risk factors. The homebirth population also had trained attendants and prenatal care. These are Dr. Mehl's findings about hospital birth outcomes compared with homebirth outcomes:

+ Three times greater likelihood of cesarean operation if a woman gave birth in a hospital

+ Twenty times more use of forceps

+ Twice as much use of oxytocin to accelerate or induce labor

+ A greater incidence of episiotomy (while at the same time having more severe tears in need of major repair)

+ Six times more infant distress in labor

+ Five times more cases of maternal high blood pressure

+ Three times greater incidence of postpartum hemorrhage

+ Four times more infection among the newborns

+ Three times more babies that needed help to begin breathing

+ The hospital group had thirty cases of birth injuries, including skull fractures, facial nerve palsies, brachial nerve injuries, and severe cephalohematomas. There were no such injuries at home.

The infant death rate was low in both situations and essentially the same. There were no maternal deaths for either home or hospital. The main differences were the significant improvements in the homebirth mothers and babies. This was true despite the fact that the homebirth statistics included those who began labor at home but ultimately needed to be transferred to the hospital.

If you're inclined to reject homebirth for fear of added risks, think again. If you and your baby are healthy and you have good prenatal care and appropriate birth attendants, there's no medical reason why you shouldn't have your baby in the security of your own home. Don't let people tell you it's irresponsible or that you're being a bad mother—I don't know of any research that will back them up.

Take to heart the following statistics from extensive studies showing that hospital birth does not necessarily mean a safe and healthy outcome.

Barbara Harper, in *Gentle Birth Choices*, reminds us that we measure the safety of birth by the "death (mortality) or illness (morbidity)" rates "during the labor and birth process and shortly thereafter." You'd think that the United States would have the best ranking in this area, but instead we have "consistently high maternal and perinatal mortality and morbidity rates compared to other industrialized countries." In fact, we were ranked twenty-third by the Population Reference Bureau in 1990—there were twenty-two other countries where it was "safer for women to give birth than in the United States."

Texas Department of Health statistics show that midwives in Texas have a lower infant mortality rate than physicians.[2] Caroline Hall Otis, in an article in the *Utne Reader*, reported the alarming statistic that the infant mortality rate for physicians is **three times** higher than the rate for midwives, i.e. the infant mortality rate for physician-attended, hospital birth is **300%** of the rate for midwife-attended home birth. She also reported that midwives, instead of physicans, attend more than 70% of the births in the five Euopean countries that have the lowest infant mortality rates.

> "In the five European countries with the lowest infant mortality rates, midwives preside at more than 70 percent of all births. More than half of all Dutch babies are born at home with midwives in attendance, and Holland's maternal and infant mortality rates are far lower than in the United States."[3]

Whether the statistics are from the United States or from other parts of the world, studies show homebirths with midwives in attendance are generally safer and have better outcomes than do hospital births attended by physicians. This final quote helps confirm this.

> "Every study that has compared midwives and obstetricians has found better outcomes for midwives for same-risk patients. In some studies, midwives actually served higher-risk populations than the physicians and still obtained lower mortalities and morbidities. The superiority and safety of midwifery for most women no longer needs to be proven. It has been well established."[4]

Birthing your baby at home is *not* a high-risk choice. It is *not* considered dangerous or neglectful on the part of the parents to plan a homebirth. It is *not* putting your baby in danger or creating complications that may harm your child. It *is* a natural instinct to have your baby in a safe and familiar environment. Isn't it good to know that what you instinctually want is actually safer for you and your baby?

Statistics and desire, although a good start, aren't all you need in order to have a successful homebirth. You also must carefully plan and prepare from the very beginning of your pregnancy. Although risk is small in a normal natural childbirth, as with anything else, there is always a chance that something can go wrong. It's important that you have a skilled person present who can anticipate the need for action, plan for it, and initiate it before an emergency situation develops.

Go With Your Instincts

When a woman is in labor, it isn't normal to go to a strange, supposedly sterile environment that in reality is rife with germs and disease. As unflattering as it may sound, we are animals, and when animals are moved during labor they either stop laboring or have their young dead. No wonder so many women who admit themselves into the hospital in early labor are diagnosed with false labor and sent home or jump started with Pitocin to "get things going." Most likely they weren't in false labor—their body stopped laboring because it instinctively knew it was no longer safe. In many cases, if not most, if the women had stayed home, labor would have continued naturally.

Maintaining personal control of your birth is the most apparent reason to have your baby at home. You're able to call the shots as long as the birth is going at a normal and natural pace. You can plan how you want to have your baby, who to have assist at your birth, and where you want to actually give birth. It's all about choice.

Choosing to have a baby at home will also ensure that you'll not be coerced into situations that aren't offered outside a hospital—for instance, medications (such as Pitocin), epidurals, and narcotics; routine procedures (such as IVs, continuous monitoring, and frequent vaginal exams), and time limits; and doctors who are rushing you or pressuring you to birth your baby sooner. When you birth your baby at home, you set the pace. You'll be monitored, but the assessments are non-intrusive and infrequent as long as the baby looks good. While in labor you'll be able to walk in the garden, soak in a tub, play the music you love, sit in your favorite chair, invite whomever you want to have present, and eat when you're hungry and need nourishment. You can cook in your own kitchen and lie in your own bed and snuggle with your partner without IVs or monitors in the way.

The people who will be attending your birth are those you'll have had an eight-month or longer relationship with, not strangers who are on call and just coming in when you're pushing, meeting you for the first time. When you choose a midwife or homebirth doctor, she will spend time with you planning your birth—going over your birth plan, visiting your home to see where you're planning to have your baby, and educating your partner about what will happen during your baby's birth. You'll be working together to make your homebirth a personal and wonderful experience.

How to Prepare for a Homebirth

Preparing for a homebirth requires careful planning and research. Begin by finding a qualified, trained midwife or a doctor who does home births (see *Chapter Two*). Large communities offer a greater selection of birth professionals to choose from. Small communities may very well offer only one choice, however, and the waiting list may be long. So as soon as you can, seek out and hire that special someone who can help you.

Interviewing a Midwife

Many homebirth midwives are certified by various qualifying bodies. Others have been practicing for years, have attended hundreds of births, and are confident in their skills. Some practitioners may have very little experience yet call themselves qualified midwives. If an emergency arises, they may not have the experience to either recognize it or act on it properly. So ask lots of questions—the wellbeing of you and your baby depends on choosing someone with the right knowledge and experience.

Here are some questions that will help you choose the best qualified midwife who is the right fit for you.

- ✦ What training does she have?
- ✦ Does she have a license or certificate from a training facility?
- ✦ What birth practitioners' organizations does she belong to?
- ✦ Does she keep her skills updated with workshops and conferences?
- ✦ How many births has she attended where she was the primary midwife?
- ✦ What do her prenatal services include?
- ✦ Has she attended high-risk births such as twins or breeches? How many?
- ✦ Does she have an assistant?
- ✦ Who is her backup if she's at another birth?
- ✦ Who is her doctor and hospital backup, and what do they think about her?
- ✦ What would make her decide to transport you to the hospital?
- ✦ Does she have good rapport with a doctor with whom she can discuss questions?
- ✦ What emergency equipment does she bring with her to a homebirth? Does she have access to oxygen?
- ✦ What kind of postpartum care does she offer, if any, or whom would she recommend to help you with your postpartum care?
- ✦ What is her philosophy about childbirth, and does it match yours?
- ✦ What is her fee?

It's a good idea to include your partner in the interviewing—both of you should feel good about the person who is going to help bring your baby into the world. You'll know when you've found the right person; both of you will feel it in your hearts.

The website *www.socialbirth.org* is a great place to find all the questions you should ask of midwives, doctors, birth attendants, and hospital personnel. Don't be afraid or shy to ask, ask, ask. Find out all you can about who will be helping with your birth.

Back to School

Your next step is to find a prenatal class geared to homebirths. These classes will not only show you good laboring techniques to help you through labor, they'll also tell you how to prepare your home, make a backup plan, and otherwise help you create a safe birth for your baby. Association for Childbirth At Home, International (ACHI), offers an excellent series of prenatal classes created by midwife and author Suzanne Arms that specifically prepares parents for a homebirth.

The best way to find prenatal classes in your community is to ask your midwife. She may teach classes herself, or she may work with a doula who teaches childbirth classes. Health food stores often have a bulletin board where you can find the names and contact information for prenatal instructors. The hospital in your area may even have a list of midwives or prenatal instructors who teach in your town. Consider searching the Internet for instructors who will suit your needs.

Plan B

One of the most important things on your to-do list is to develop a plan in case things don't go the way you expect. A backup plan lets everyone know what you want to do, where you want to go, and who you want to assist you if you have problems in labor and must be transported to the hospital.

Arrange for a doctor who will attend you at the hospital if there are complications and you must be transported. You wouldn't want to show up needing immediate medical attention and be assigned to an on-call doctor you have never met. Your midwife probably knows a doctor or two who will back her up. Make appointments with them and interview them, then choose the one who will work best with you.

Not only is it your responsibility to find a doctor who will care for you and your baby if necessary, it's also your responsibility to find a hospital or clinic that won't turn you away when you need medical assistance. If you live in a large city with several hospitals and you're not in an emergency situation and you have no insurance a hospital can direct you to another facility. So be sure this is arranged months before your baby is due so the doctor will get to know you and understand your desire to have your baby as naturally as possible even if you're in the hospital.

Part of your backup plan is knowing what situation your midwife would consider an emergency and what would cause her to decide to transport you to the hospital or clinic. Sort all of this out and make your agreements before the birth so there will be no arguing or misunderstandings if she wants you transported. An important point you must agree to: if you decide to go to the hospital—even for no apparent reason—then *you go to the hospital.* I've attended several births where, for no apparent reason, the mom said she needed to go to the hospital. Lo and behold, an unforeseen complication truly existed that had to be dealt with. So trust your instincts— they're working overtime in labor.

Post a list of phone numbers near your primary telephone. This is also a good place to keep a map to the hospital/clinic, insurance information, and your medical records. Make sure there's always gas in the car and babysitters lined up if you have children you'll be leaving at home.

Important Phone Numbers

Doctor: _____

Midwife: _____

Doula: _____

Other Attendants

Babysitter: _____

Hospital: _____

Maternity Ward: _____

Emergency Room: _____

Back up Doctor: _____

Taxi: _____

Things to Keep at the Ready

✦ A small suitcase packed with personal belongings:

— toothbrush, hairbrush, shampoo, makeup

— your own nightgown

— clothes to come home in

— an outfit for the baby, with a hat and blankets.

✦ Car seat for the baby. Hospitals won't discharge a baby without a car seat to take him home in.

✦ Favorite music you would be using at home for the birth. Though it'll be an emergency or failure to progress that brings you in, there still may be some time until the birth, and music will help you cope.

Prepare Your Nest

Now you have a midwife, a doula, prenatal classes, a backup plan, and a healthy pregnancy. It's time to collect your supplies and find out what to do with them.

Look at your home from the perspective of a birthing woman, and decide which room you want to have your baby in. Set up your home accordingly. Some choose to have their baby in a spare bedroom so they can set it up early. Some place a spare bed in the living room where there is more room to move around. Others choose to have their babies in the bed where the baby was conceived. This takes a little extra work because you'll be preparing the bed while you're laboring. In any case you'll want a few things on hand so you won't have to worry about them while you're in labor.

For a first-time mom, labor usually lasts an average of 12 to 18 hours. Now's the time to gather some items to ease you through the hours. Go through your CDs and set aside some favorites, or pull out a favorite movie. Shop for candles and incense, oils and lotions, for those wonderful massages you'll be entitled to, and some bubble bath or nice bath oils for laboring in the tub. During early labor, ask someone to go to the store for fresh fruit or a treat you especially enjoy. And have lots of bottled water ready in the fridge.

All the laundry you'll be using for the big day must be sterilized in advance. Don't panic—this task is much easier than it sounds. Generally, you'll need:

+ two sets of sheets with pillow cases,

+ four or five towels and wash cloths,

+ an outfit for the baby,

+ diapers (disposable or cloth),

+ something comfortable for you to put on after you have your baby, and

+ a sheet cut into quarters for extra cloths to use during the birth.

To sterilize these items, simply wash them in hot water and dry them thoroughly using your dryer's hottest setting. With clean hands place the items in a new large-size plastic bag, seal it, then store it away for the birth day. You can do this ahead of time, but the contents must be rewashed and dried if you don't use them within seven days.

When the time comes to prepare your birthing bed, you'll use both sets of sheets. Make up your bed with the first set as usual, then cover it completely with a clean shower curtain or a plastic drop cloth. Make up the bed with the second set of sheets over the drop cloth—this is the set you'll labor in. After you've had your baby, have someone remove the used top set of sheets and the drop cloth, and you'll be left with a nicely made up bed with clean sheets and minimum hassle.

Birth Day

Now that everything is ready for your homebirth, start taking it easy. During the last couple of weeks before your due date, try to take a nap every afternoon. This isn't as far fetched as it sounds—you'll be sleepier than usual, and your body and your baby will welcome some extra snooze time. Also, because most labors begin in the evening hours, you'll be more rested.

So contractions have started. Time-wise, you're in the safety zone—38 to 42 weeks pregnant—and everything is ready. You should have finished your last prenatal class several weeks ago, and your birth plans, backup plans, phone numbers, and so forth are where they should be. Everyone is on standby, ready and waiting, and you couldn't be calmer, right?

Now is the time to give your midwife a call. She needs to know the minute you start showing signs of labor so she can cancel any other plans and rearrange her priorities. She'll come to your home to see how you're doing and drop off some of her equipment. She may or may not check your cervix, depending on how active your labor is. If you both decide that you're in very early labor and you feel comfortable about her leaving, she may go back home and organize things for her upcoming absence. Meanwhile, you'll casually labor with friends or family until she is needed. Be sure to call her if your membranes break—she'll want to check you to ensure there are no problems with the umbilical cord.

Call everyone who is going to be a part of your birth and tell them when you would like them to come. Then, take a nap, or at least lie down and rest as quietly as you can before you start active labor.

When you're up again, go for a walk, putter around the garden, bake some cookies, make some tea—whatever will keep you vertical. Gravity helps move your baby down into position. When your labor becomes regular, meaning that stronger contractions are coming closer together, call your midwife again. This time when she comes she'll check your cervix, help set up your birth bed, and probably settle in for the duration.

Throughout your labor your midwife will check your baby's heart rate every hour until your cervix is 8 centimeters dilated. Then she'll check you every thirty minutes. She'll help you settle on a breathing technique, check your cervix when she sees significant changes in your labor, remind you to keep yourself well nourished, support your decisions, and incorporate and support your partner and family throughout the birth process. When you're ready to have your baby she'll help you try various positions, advise you how to push most effectively, and eventually "catch" your baby!

After you have your baby your midwife will help you initiate breastfeeding. She'll clean up, settle things down, and stay with you for a couple of hours to make sure you and baby are doing fine. In the following days she'll visit you frequently and call you to ensure you feel comfortable and at ease in your new role as a mother.

Forrest's Birth

The following birth story will give you an idea about what homebirth can be like. This birth was one of my favorites I attended as a midwife. I admired how well Matthew and Janis worked together and how loving their family was.

I met Janis and Matthew through Dr. Una Jean Sayles after they asked her to attend their homebirth with a midwife in attendance. We talked on the phone for more than an hour about what they wanted for their birth and what other options they had considered. As it turned out, we all agreed and got along very well.

The couple was in the fifth month of their first pregnancy and were eager to learn all they could. Their decision to birth their baby at home was based on experiences their friends had had having their babies in hospitals. The couple had been told how their friends didn't get what they wanted, how plans were interrupted by interventions they didn't anticipate, and in general how disappointed everyone was with the entire experience. Janis and Matthew wanted to have more control over their special day, so after carefully researching their options, they chose to birth their baby at home with Dr. Sayles and me.

Janis and Matthew signed up for the six-week Wednesday night prenatal classes that I was teaching in my home at the time. The classes covered subjects such as nutrition, stages of pregnancy and what to expect, choosing birth attendants and physicians, breathing and relaxation techniques, and how to prepare for a homebirth. I discussed what to expect during labor and the baby's birth and what supplies to have on hand and how to prepare them. Although my primary focus is on birthing babies at home, I also prepare couples for the possibility of being transferred to the hospital, how to devise their backup plan, and how to choose a physician who will work with them. I emphasize what their rights are and what help is available to them when they get there.

I visited Janis and Matthew at their home twice before their baby's birth. The first time, my long-time midwifery mentor, Sandra Botting, and I went together so we all could get acquainted, see where the couple wanted to birth, and get a feeling for what would be ideal for them. During the second visit I gave the couple a detailed list of things to have available for the birth.

Two weeks later, at three o'clock in the afternoon, Matthew called to say Janis had been having contractions irregularly since the middle of the previous night. Her membranes were intact, and contractions were about seven to ten minutes apart. I went to their house to help set up their bedroom and check Janis's cervix. She was 3 centimeters dilated. I called Dr. Sayles to give her a heads-up on Janis's progress and tell her Janis was handling her labor well. I stayed with Janis and Matthew for a while and then, seeing that they were doing so well on their own, I headed home to arrange for babysitting and prepare for a long night.

At 10 p.m. Matthew called again and told me Janis's contractions were about five minutes apart and regular. She was having trouble talking through them, which told me she was really starting to "cook." I called Sandy and arranged for her to meet me at Matthew and Janis's, and then called Dr. Sayles, who would join us when Janis reached 9 or 10 centimeters dilation or started feeling the need to push. I gathered my birth bag and headed over to their house.

I arrived about twenty minutes before Sandy and found Janis in the living room, rocking in her favorite chair and in the middle of a contraction. She was working pretty hard at keeping focused, and Matthew was kneeling on the floor in front of her helping her breathe. Janis's mother and sister were puttering around in the kitchen, making raspberry leaf tea and trying to stay out of Janis and Matthew's way.

I made sure everything was where it should be in the bedroom and then began sterilizing some of the equipment I had brought with me. Sandy arrived, and after introducing herself to Janis's family she helped arrange things. We continued to check the baby's heart rate every thirty minutes and kept a detailed record of mom's progress. Matthew and Janis labored together beautifully. He stroked her head, wiped her brow, breathed with her during her contractions, and catered to her every whim. Sandy and I hung back and gave them a chance to labor together in privacy.

At about one o'clock in the morning, after Janis had been in the bathtub a couple of times and had walked around in the backyard, her contractions changed. She was feeling the need to push with them and felt added pressure in her rectum. I checked her, and sure enough she was fully dilated and ready to push her baby out. I called Dr. Sayles and then helped Janis move to the bedroom where she wanted to have her baby. Dr. Sayles arrived soon after, set up her equipment, checked the baby's heart rate, and confirmed that Janis was indeed fully dilated.

Sometimes a midwife can feel like a third wheel because the couple is working so well together. This was one of those times, and it was beautiful to witness. Janis chose to start pushing using Matthew as support. Matthew sat on the bed so the headboard supported his back. Janis sat between his legs with her back to his chest so he could wipe her brow, stroke her head, and cradle her tenderly between pushes.

In anticipation of baby's debut, we dimmed the lights and turned the heat up to 80 degrees for his comfort. Dr. Sayles kneeled next to Janis, taking it all in while I sat at the foot of the bed, gloved, giving Janis instructions about how to push effectively. After about forty-five minutes I could see the top of the baby's head. Sandy was gathering warmed blankets for the baby, a suction bulb syringe, a cord clamp, and a bowl for the placenta. I started lubricating the perineum with warmed oil to help it stretch.

When the baby's head started to crown, just before he was born, I told Janis to stop pushing with her contractions and just start panting heavily. I asked her to push between contractions so I could help control how fast the head was delivered and spare her from tearing. Slowly, Janis pushed her baby's head out while I supported the perineum and gently put pressure on the head to stop it from shooting out. After the head eased out, I checked to see if his umbilical cord was wrapped around his neck; it wasn't. As nature designed it, he turned so his shoulders could emerge. As Janis gently pushed, the shoulders came out one at a time. Then I carefully guided her new son out onto the warmed blankets. Forrest was born at 2:45 a.m. Because Matthew was cradling Janis and couldn't reach the cord to cut it, he asked her mother if she would do the honors, which she did.

I checked Forrest's breathing and his heart rate at the base of the umbilical cord, then quickly dried him while I placed him on his mommy's tummy. He was beautiful! He pinked up immediately after he was born and had a good vigorous cry. His daddy was also crying, and Janis was laughing as she hugged their son. Off to the side grandma and auntie were hugging each other, tears running down their faces. Dr. Sayles checked the baby more thoroughly while mom held him, and then she checked to see if there were any tears in Janis's perineum. It was intact. Janis expelled the placenta without complications.

Expelling the placenta takes patience and time. An impressive natural process happens after the baby is born to help expel the placenta. Baby first lies on mommy's tummy with his eyes closed. In about five minutes he opens his eyes and quietly looks around. About twenty minutes later the baby starts to root, bobbing his head on mommy's chest with his mouth open looking for his first meal. If mom offers her breast the baby will latch on and start sucking. The mom's uterus reacts to the sucking and immediately contracts, expelling the placenta without difficulty. This process can't be rushed—complications could arise, such as tearing of the placenta, or if the cord is pulled it can break, causing the mom to bleed uncontrollably.

Once the placenta was expelled, Dr. Sayles checked it to ensure it was intact and that there were no pieces left inside mom that could cause hemorrhage. Then she checked the fundus (uterus) by pressing on Janis's lower abdomen to see if it was firm, about the size of a large grapefruit, and not filling with blood.

The baby was checked again for heart rate, breathing rate, color, muscle tone, and reflexes. All was well, so Sandy and I cleaned up. Dr. Sayles thoroughly examined both mom and baby, made follow-up appointments for both of them, and then headed home.

After Janis breastfed, Matthew held Forrest while we helped mom into the shower, changed her bedding, got her into clean jammies, checked her bleeding, and tucked her into bed with Matthew and their new son. Grandma, auntie, Sandy, and I said our goodnights and quietly left the new family. The couple had been in control of everything, had done all they had wanted to do during labor and their baby's birth, and everyone had come to them for the event. It was a beautiful birth.

I visited the little family twice a day for a week to make sure breastfeeding was going well and that their son was thriving. Then I visited once a day for the next week to make sure Janis had no problems and to answer all her questions.

A Little Help From Your Friends

I hope this chapter has helped you get your plans started if you have decided to birth your baby at home. Plenty of websites and books are available to help inform and inspire you further. Be sure to do your research and follow up with good prenatal care and planning. Here is a list of excellent reading. Any of these sources will help you decide if homebirth is right for you.

1. Diana Korte, *A Good Birth, A Safe Birth: Choosing and Having the Childbirth Experience You Want*, Harvard Common Press, 1992

2. Elizabeth Davis, *Heart & Hands*: *A Midwife's Guide to Pregnancy and Birth*, Third edition, Celestial Arts, 1997

3. Sheila Kitzinger, *Birth At Home* [now titled *Homebirth*], Penguin, 1979

4. Nial Ettinghausen, *Childbirth At Its Best: The Ettinghausen Method*, Candor Pub. Co., 1980

5. Suzanne Arms, *Immaculate Deception*, Bergin & Garvey, 1985

6. Barbara Harper, Suzanne Arms, *Gentle Birth Choices: A Guide to Making Informed Decisions About Birthing Centers, Birth Attendants, Water Birth, Home Birth, Hospital Birth*, Healing Art Press, 1994

7. Deborah Sullivan and Rose Weitz, *Labor Pains: Modern Midwives and Homebirth*, Yale University Press, 1988

8. *Midwifery Today*, P.O. Box 2672, Eugene, OR 97402, quarterly magazine, email newsletter, quarterly newsletters

9. Carl Jones, *Mind Over Labor*, Viking Penguin, 1988

10. *Mothering*, P.O. Box 1690, Santa Fe, NM 87504, quarterly magazine

11. David & Lee Stewart, eds., *Safe Alternatives in Childbirth*, NAPSAC Intl

12. Rahima Baldwin, *Special Delivery*, Celestial Arts, 1979

13. Ina May Gaskin, *Spiritual Midwifery*, fourth ed., The Book Publishing Co., 2002

14. *The Birth Gazette*, 42 Summertown, TN 38483, quarterly magazine

15. Doris Haire, *The Cultural Warping of Childbirth*, International Childbirth Education Association, 1972

16. David Stewart, *The Five Standards for Safe Childbearing*, NAPSAC Reproductions, 1981

16. *The NAPSAC Directory*, Rt.1, Box 646, P.O. Box 267, Marble Hill, MO 63764

17. Ina May Gaskin, *Ina May's Guide to Childbirth*, Bantam Books, 2003

Homebirth

Okay, you've read the homebirth chapter, you've consulted with a physician or midwife and found you and your baby are doing great and your pregnancy is right on track. This worksheet will now help you gather up everything that you'll need to have your baby at home.

First, get those phone numbers and have them by your phone: These include the people that you have already chosen from the *Hiring the Help* section of this book.

Midwife _____ Phone _____

Address _____

Her Back-up _____ Phone _____

Address _____

Physician _____ Phone _____

Address _____

His Back-up _____ Phone _____

Address _____

Doula _____ Phone _____

Address _____

Her Back-up _____ Phone _____

Address _____

Babysitter (If you have other siblings to watch) _____

Phone _____

Address: _____

People you want to have with you

Name: _____ Phone: _____

Name: _____ Phone: _____

Name: _____ Phone: _____

Emergency numbers

Hospital: _____ Maternity Ward: _____

Emergency Ward: _____ Taxi: _____

Getting Ready

	Yes	No
1. I will be taking prenatal classes.	❏	❏

If yes, they will be provided by:

❏ my midwife

❏ my hospital

❏ Bradley

❏ ACHI

❏ Lamaze

❏ other _____

2. In case I have to go to the hospital, I'll have the following ready:

❏ A small suitcase or travel bag packed with:

❏ toothbrush

❏ hair products

❏ nightgown

❏ clothes to come home in

❏ baby clothes

❏ favorite music or DVDs, magazines, etc.

❏ A car-seat (you can't leave the hospital without one)

3. I have decided to have my baby in the following:

❏ living room

❏ bedroom

❏ spare bedroom

❏ bathtub

❏ other (this could even be at another home) _____

4. I'll have the following personal things ready for my labor at home:

❑ candles

❑ music

❑ favorite movies

❑ beverages

❑ snacks

❑ massage oils

❑ bubble bath

❑ camera(s), with lots of film and batteries

❑ other _____

5. I'll have the following supplies ready for the actual birth:

❑ two sets of sterilized sheets with pillow cases

❑ four or five bath towels and wash clothes

❑ a new soft plastic painter's drop-cloth

❑ a sheet cut into rags to use during the birth

❑ diapers

❑ an outfit for the baby

❑ a change of clothes for myself

That's about it. There isn't much, since your midwife or doula will help you with a lot of things before you have your baby.

One more thing: Please mail me at Breck@writeme.com after your special day—I want to know how it went!

8

Waterbirths:
From Newborn
Breathing
to Hospital
Protocols

✦

*Getting Into Hot Water
with Barbara Harper, RN*

"If you obey all the rules you miss all the fun."
— Katherine Hepburn

Barbara Harper, RN is the founder and President of Global Maternal/Child Health Association and current director of the Waterbirth International Resource and Referral Service. A childbirth educator, doula, and traditional midwife, Barbara has spent 22 years in nursing. She is the author of *Gentle Birth Choices*, and producer of the *Gentle Birth Choices* video.

When I asked Barbara for some information on waterbirths for my book, she kindly sent me this article that she had written for *Midwifery Today* magazine (Issue 54, Summer 2000) and graciously gave me permission to share it with you. It is reprinted here in its entirety as Chapter 8. Enjoy.

Waterbirth is simple

Within the simplicity of water, labor and birth lies a complexity of questions, choices, opinions, research data, women's experience, and practitioner observations.

As more hospitals within the United States examine waterbirth and create programs to support the use of water for labor and birth, newspaper reporters latch onto the sensationalism of this simple option and publish stories of successful waterbirths in local publications. Each reporter does their best to simplify waterbirth and at the same time answer the most common questions. Each story shows a happy, beaming mother, a quiet, peaceful baby, and a proud father, who usually successfully set up a portable birth pool. The surprise headlines, like "Watery birth," "Baby's birth goes swimmingly," or "Junior makes a splashy entrance," are countered with the simple stories of couples who have made this decision for themselves and are proud of it.

How does the baby breathe during a waterbirth?

There are several factors that prevent a baby from inhaling water at the time of birth. These inhibitory factors are normally present in all newborns. The baby in utero is oxygenated through the umbilical cord via the placenta, but practices for future air breathing by moving his intercostal muscles and diaphragm in a regular and rhythmic pattern from about 10 weeks gestation on. The lung fluids that are present are produced in the lungs and similar chemically to gastric fluids. These fluids come out into the mouth and are normally swallowed by the fetus. There is very little inspiration of amniotic fluid in utero. Twenty-four to forty-eight hours before the onset of spontaneous labor the fetus experiences a notable increase in the Prostaglandin E2 levels from the placenta, which cause a slowing down or stopping of the fetal breathing movements (FBM).[1] With the work of the musculature of the diaphragm and intercostal muscles suspended, there is more blood flow to vital organs, including the brain. You can see the decrease in FBM on a biophysical profile, as you normally see the fetus moving these muscles about 40 percent of the time. When the baby is born and the prostaglandin level is still high, the baby's muscles for breathing simply don't work, thus engaging the first inhibitory response.

A second inhibitory response is that babies are born experiencing acute hypoxia, or lack of oxygen. It is a built-in response to the birth process. Hypoxia causes apnea and swallowing, not breathing or gasping. If the fetus were experiencing severe and prolonged lack of oxygen, it may then gasp as soon as it was born, possibly inhaling water into the lungs.[2] If the baby were in trouble during the labor, there would be wide variations noted in the fetal heart rate, usually resulting in prolonged bradycardia, which would cause the practitioner to ask the mother to leave the bath prior to the baby's birth.

Another factor that is thought by many to inhibit the newborn from initiating the breathing response while in water is the temperature differential. The temperature of the water is so close to that of the maternal temperature that it prevents any detection of change within the newborn. This is an area for reconsideration after increasing reports of births taking place in the oceans, both now and in eras past. Ocean temperatures are certainly not as high as maternal body temperature and yet the babies that are born in these environments are reported to be just fine. The lower water temperatures do not stimulate the baby to breathe while immersed.

One more factor that most people do not consider, but is vital to the whole waterbirth and aspiration issue, is that water is a hypotonic solution and lung fluids present in the fetus are hypertonic. So, even if water were to travel in past the larynx, it could not pass into the lungs because hypertonic solutions are denser and prevent hypotonic solutions from merging or coming into their presence.

The last important inhibitory factor is the Dive Reflex, which revolves around the larynx. The larynx is covered all over with chemoreceptors, or taste buds. The larynx has five times as many as taste buds as the whole surface of the tongue. So when a solution hits the back of the throat, passing the larynx, the taste buds interpret what substance it is, the glottis automatically closes, and the solution is then swallowed, not inhaled.[3] God built this autonomic reflex into all newborns to assist with breastfeeding; it is present until about the age of six to eight months, when it mysteriously disappears. The newborn is very intelligent and can detect what substance is in its throat. It can differentiate between amniotic fluid, water, and cow's milk or human milk. The human infant will swallow and breathe differently when feeding on cow's milk or breast milk due to the Dive Reflex.

All of these factors combine to prevent a newborn that is born into water from taking a breath until he is lifted up into the air.

What does happen to initiate the breath in the newborn?

As soon as the newborn senses a change in the environment from the water into the air, there is a complex chain of chemical, hormonal, and physical responses, all resulting in the baby breathing. Water-born babies are slower to initiate this response because their whole body is exposed to the air at the same time, not just the caput or head as in a dry birth. Many midwives report that water babies stay just a little bit bluer longer, but their tone and alertness are just fine. It has even been suggested that water-born babies be given the first APGAR scoring at one minute thirty seconds, not at one minute, due to this adjustment.

There are several things that happen all at once for the baby. The shunts in the heart are closed, fetal circulation turns to newborn circulation, the lungs experience oxygen for the first time, and the umbilical cord is stretched, causing the umbilical arteries to close down. Nursing and medical schools taught their students for years that the first breath was dependent on the pressure of the passage through the birth canal and then a reflexive opening of the compressed chest creating a vacuum. But now we know that action has no bearing on newborn breathing whatsoever. There is no vacuum created. The newborn that is born into water is protected by all the inhibitory mechanisms mentioned above, and is suspended and waiting to be lifted up out of the water and into mother's waiting arms.

All the fluids that are present in the lung alveoli are automatically pushed out into the vascular system from the pressure of pulmonary circulation, thus increasing blood volume for the newborn by 1/5, or 20 percent. The lymphatic system absorbs the rest of the fluids through the interstitial spaces in the lung tissue. The increase of blood volume is vital for the baby's health. It takes about six hours for all the lung fluids to disappear.[4]

When we look back at the analysis of the statistics of babies born in water it proves that these inhibitory factors are more than theories. A study conducted in England between 1994 and 1996, and published in 1999, reports on the outcomes of 4032 births in water. Perinatal mortality was 1.2 per 1000, but no deaths were attributed to birth in the water. Two babies were admitted to special care for possible water aspiration.[5] From 1985 to 1999, it is estimated that there have been well over 150,000 cases of waterbirth worldwide. There are no valid reports of infant deaths due to water aspiration or inhalation.

Although in the early days of waterbirth a baby was reported as dying from being born in the water, this particular newborn death was caused not by aspiration, but by asphyxiation due to leaving the baby under the water for more than fifteen minutes after the full body was born. At some point the placenta detached from the wall of the uterus and stopped the flow of oxygen to the baby. When the baby was taken out of the water, it did not begin breathing and could not be revived. On autopsy the baby was reported to have no water in the lungs and its death was attributed to asphyxia.[6]

This is the reason that we bring babies up out of the water within the first few moments after birth. Some people have commented on the long time that some babies remain in the water in the film *Water Babies: The Aquanatal Experience in Ostend.* Video tape is deceiving, but so are our senses. When timed, the film sequence is only forty-seven seconds, but when viewers are asked to judge how long the sequence of immersion for the baby really is, reports range anywhere from one minute to five minutes.

Bringing a baby out of the water too quickly can be just as traumatic, but it can also lead to either torn or broken cords. This has been reported by a number of midwives and doctors.[7] If the practitioner is not looking for a torn cord, the possibility of the baby needing a transfusion increases. Torn or broken cords can be avoided by bringing baby out of the water slowly and gently. Mothers who desire to pick up their own babies also need to be reminded to not do it too quickly.

The inability to accurately assess blood loss in the water is a reason that some midwives have stated for either not "allowing" the birth to take place in the water or asking mother to get out right away after the baby is born. But blood loss assessment is easy to judge after a few births. Garland and Jones report in a review of waterbirths at Maidstone Hospital in Kent, England, that the midwives are much better at judging and reporting blood loss in the water after experiencing over 500 births.[8] A useful key to judge post-partum hemorrhage is to watch how dark the water is getting. Can you still assess skin color of the mother's thighs even though there is blood in the water? A few drops of water in a birth pool diffuses and causes it to change color. A waterproof flashlight comes in handy at this point. Dropping a flashlight onto the bottom of the birth pool allows you to look for bleeding as well as meconium during the birth. It also helps you spot floating debris and remove it.

Won't the mother get an infection?

There are still hospitals that restrict a woman from laboring in the water if her membranes are ruptured. This is totally absurd based on the current and past literature. There is no evidence of an increase in infectious morbidity with or without ruptured membranes for women who labor and/or birth in water.[9,10] The oldest reference that researches the possibility of infection during a bath is mentioned in a 1960 American Journal of OB/GYN. Dr. Siegel posed the question, "Does bath water enter the vagina?" In his experiment he placed sterile cotton tampons into thirty women and then asked them to bath in iodinated water for a minimum of fifteen minutes. In all cases, when the tampons were removed, there was no iodine present.[11] His conclusion states, "We can now stop restricting women from bathing in the later stages of pregnancy and labor." Laboring mothers have an advantage: when the baby is descending and moving out. Nothing is moving up and in.

Things that we put into laboring vaginas may cause an increase in infections, such as probes, fingers, amnihooks, scalp hooks, etc. Janet Rush, RN, and her Canadian group of investigators have conducted the only randomized controlled trial of the effects of water labor. They reported that there were no differences noted in the low rates of maternal and newborn signs of infection in women with ruptured membranes.[12]

Infection control, especially in a hospital setting, requires diligence and the following of strict protocols between and during births. Cleaning and maintaining all equipment used for a waterbirth will prevent the spread of infection. In a random study conducted at the Oregon Health Science University Hospital in 1999, cultures were done from the portable jetted birth pool before, during, and after birth, as well as from the fill hose and water tap source. In no instances did bacteria culture from the birth pool, but the water tap did culture Pseudomonas.[13] In a British study of 541 water labors no serious infections were reported during the three-year period of data gathering. Again, Pseudomonas aeruginosa was the only persistent bacteria discovered in two babies who tested positive from ear swabs. No treatment was necessary.[14]

Some parents are concerned about mother-to-mother infections or contamination from viruses such as HIV or hepatitis. But there is no reason to restrict an HIV positive mother from laboring or giving birth in water; all evidence indicates that the HIV virus cannot live in a warm water environment.[15] Universal precautions still need to be adhered to, of course, and proper cleaning of all the equipment after the birth needs to be carried out.

Using disposable liners has become the norm with portable birth pools, but attention must also be paid to proper cleaning of drain pumps, hoses, filter nets, taps, and any other items that are reused from one birth to the next. The issue of cleaning the jets of permanently-installed baths has generated some concern and discussion over the past few years. Many hospitals remodeled their labor units in the late eighties or early nineties, installing whirlpool baths. These baths are great for women in labor, but often are not deep enough, or are situated within very small bathroom spaces, boxed in and making birth in them difficult in all respects. The protocol for cleaning jetted tubs is simply to completely clean the tub with a quaternary ammonium solution, refill with water, and add some kind of brominating agent to circulate through the jet system for a minimum of ten minutes.[16] A number of hospitals report that they use a half cup of powdered dishwashing crystals, such as Cascade, and it works fine. Lynn Springer, RN, the perinatal coordinator for St. Elizabeth Hospital in Red Bluff, California, chose to install a beautiful corner Jacuzzi-brand jetted bath on her unit in 1995. They routinely performed monthly cultures of the bath and the jets throughout five years of their water birth program without any significant bacterial growth. They follow the above-mentioned cleaning protocol and report over 1000 water labors and 400 births in water.[17]

When should the mother enter the bath?

Many hospitals use the 5-centimeter rule—only allowing mothers to enter the bath when they are in active labor and dilated to more than 5 centimeters. There is some physiological data that supports this rule, but each and every situation must be evaluated and then judged accordingly.

Some mothers find a bath in early labor useful for its calming effect and to determine if labor has actually started.[18] But the water sometimes has the effect of slowing or stopping labor if used too early. On the other hand, if contractions are strong and regular with either a small amount of dilation or none at all, a bath might be in order to help the mother to relax enough to facilitate the dilation. It has been suggested that the bath be used in a "trial of water" for at least one hour and allow the mother to judge its effectiveness. Women report that often the contractions seem to space out or become less effective if they enter the bath too soon, thus requiring them to leave. Then again, midwives report that some women can go from 1 cm to complete dilation within the first hour or two of immersion.

Deep immersion seems to be a key factor. If the pool or bath is not deep enough, at least providing water up to breast level and completely covering the belly, then the benefits of the bath may be less noticeable. The warm water will still provide comfort and the mother will benefit from being upright, in control and drug free, but full immersion adds more physiological responses, the most notable being a redistribution of blood volume, which stimulates the release of oxytocin and vasopressin.[19] Vasopressin can also work to increase the levels of oxytocin.[20] The immediate pain reduction upon entering the bath is quite noticeable. It is what I refer to as "the ahh effect." The smile, the sound, and the inner peace that mothers display are unmistakable. This response can happen at any point in the labor, but most notably when contractions are long and strong and close together. Some midwives who assume that there is little or no progress in dilation because the mother is not displaying any outward signs of discomfort are often surprised to find rapid dilation in the first hour of immersion. Having experienced a waterbirth myself, I can verify the incredible difference in perception of pain from the room to the water. When I am with a woman in labor I generally assess her pain on a scale of 1 to 10 before she enters the bath. Most report at least a 6 or greater. Then, after no less than half an hour, I will make another assessment. The second subjective answer, of course, varies from person to person, but the typical response is 2 to 4. The mother is experiencing more than the sum of her physiological responses to warm-water immersion. Most women feel inherently safe in the water.

The water creates a wonderful barrier to the outside world. It becomes her nest, her cave, her own "womb with a view." If the pool is large enough to include her partner or husband, it then becomes an intimate place for the two of them to labor together and experience the love dance of birth. If the midwife or physician wants to do a vaginal examination while the mother is in the water, it is much easier for the mother to refuse. Her mobility allows her to move quickly to the other side of the pool. Vaginal exams can be easily done in the water, but for universal precautions to be maintained, long shoulder-length gloves need to be worn.

The control that women gain by being able to move freely in the water often aids them in assessing their own progress either through feeling the movements of the baby more intensively or actually being able to examine themselves internally. Women report that the water intensifies the connection with the baby at the same time that it reduces the pain. They can feel the baby move, descend, and push through the birth canal. The prospect of the midwife becoming an active observer increases as mothers assume more and more responsibility for the birth and have the ease of mobility in the water. For many reasons, including reducing the risk of infection for the provider, many midwives suggest a hands-off birth for the mother. The water slows the crowning and offers its own perineal support.[21] This "minimal-touch" approach also gives the mother a greater sense of controlling her own birth.

Perineal trauma is reported to be generally less severe, with more intact perineums for multips, but about the same frequency of tears for primips in or out of the water in some of the literature.[22,23] One of the best benefits of waterbirth is the zero episiotomy rate that is reported throughout the literature. Rosenthal mentions that episiotomies can be done, but no one else offers this suggestion. The combination of being upright, having the mother in a good physiological position to birth her baby, giving her the freedom of control, and not telling her to push when her body is not indicating it, all contribute to better perineal outcomes.

Midwives have a great deal of influence over the outcome of a birth, from the suggestions they make to a laboring mother to how they handle potential complications. There is an interesting phenomenon within the waterbirth movement that deserves some discussion. When a mother is laboring undisturbed, as Odent has written and lectured, she will find her own place and time of birth, whether that place is the bathroom floor, under the piano, on the bed, or in the bath. If practitioners remain silent observers to the process, the baby is born wherever it happens. But if the mother has stated her intentions for a waterbirth and the necessary arrangements have been made to have water available, is the midwife influencing the mother by reminding her as second stage approaches or in the middle of second stage that the bath is ready and waiting if she wants to get back in? In observing the statistics that Waterbirth International gathers from midwives and doctors on waterbirth, it is hard not to notice the variance from practice to practice. Those midwives that report an 80- to 90-percent waterbirth rate are usually set up with either a birth center facility that uses easily accessible bathtubs, or every single one of their home birth clients rent or use portable birth pools. When the mother is in the midst of her subconscious birth responses, if someone tells her that the bath is ready and waiting, she often will immediately dash for the pool and climb in, even in the pushing stage. On occasion she simply states that nothing in heaven and earth can move her beyond where she is.

A midwife's or physician's hesitancy for using water for birth can also be felt by the mother and she often acquiesces just to make her practitioner feel more comfortable, instead of following her own instincts and staying in the water. Many women in hospitals get out of the pool because they don't want to get their midwives "in trouble" by insisting on giving birth in water. And in the reverse, midwives often must insist that mother get out of the pool because protocols have not been set up for birth, or the practitioner is just not comfortable with the process. The decision to birth in the water should be left up to the mother, but based on sound advice and assessment of fetal wellbeing by the practitioner. The mother who presents prenatally and is insistent that she is going to have a water birth no matter what, is usually destined to birth anywhere but the birth pool. I seriously counsel women who are taking on the system to evaluate their reasons for wanting to birth in water. If they are seeking to avoid pain only, that is a serious red flag and needs to be addressed on many different levels. If they have experienced one birth already and know what to expect and are looking for a better birth experience, then they are usually open to using the water to be in greater control and seeing how they feel at the time of birth. Flexibility is always required in birth, but especially for those women who add the element of water. In my own case, the first time I felt that I wanted to birth in water because it was the best thing I could do for my baby. I hear many women say this and that is a reasonable motivation. But the benefit that women derive from being in the water and gaining control over their experience is passed on to the baby. It is better to focus on the mother and what she needs. For my second waterbirth, no one could keep me out of the water. I was completely focused on my experience and not the baby's. Fathers will often call our office and make all the arrangements for the birth pool rental. On occasion that is because the dad wants his baby to be born in water and no other place, not taking into account what the mother really wants. Usually it all works out just fine, but occasionally it can influence the outcome of the labor.

Protocols

Protocols differ from place to place, but as more experience with waterbirth emerges, we find that some previous reasons for asking a woman to leave the bath prior to birth are no longer hard and fast.

- ✦ Meconium used to mean that the mother would have to leave the pool to birth her baby on the bed to facilitate immediate suctioning. This requirement has relaxed a bit as it has been seen that meconium washes off the face of the baby and even comes out of the nares and mouth while the baby is still under the water. DeLee suctioning can still be accomplished as soon as the baby is up in mother's arms.

- ✦ Tight nuchal cords were a reason to ask mother to stand for the birth so that the practitioner could cut the cord and then catch the baby. Now, the universal practice is to not even feel for a cord in a waterbirth unless there has been a very slow second stage and you are afraid of cord compression. No attempt is made to clamp and cut the cord. The body is birthed and then the cord is unwrapped. It is amazing to watch a baby somersault and begin to unwrap its own cord in the expanse of the birth pool.

✦ Breech position was definitely a reason for a more controlled birth or even an automatic cesarean section. But there are practitioners throughout the world who recognize that there is increased safety for the baby if it is born in water. The most experienced doctor that we know of is Hermann Ponette, an obstetrician who practices at H. Surreys Hospital in Ostend, Belgium. He has attended well over 2000 waterbirths, including breeches and twins. He uses a frank breech position as an *indication* for a waterbirth.[24] There are other reports of a few hospitals in the U.S. attending breech waterbirths and approximately 50 reported breech births in water at home.[25]

✦ Shoulder dystocia is considered an obstetric or midwifery emergency by most practitioners. Protocols require mothers who are anticipating large babies to leave the bath. Now there is a growing body of experience that suggests that shoulder dystocia, a difficult delivery situation where the shoulders get stuck in the birth canal after the baby's head is delivered, can be managed easier in the pool. Canadian midwife Gloria Lemay has written a protocol for management of shoulder dystocia in the water. It appears that tight shoulders happen more often because of practitioners or moms trying to push before the baby fully rotates. Position changes in the water are so much easier to effect and the mother doesn't panic but remains calm. A quick switch to hands and knees or even to standing up with one foot up on the edge of the pool if shoulders are really tight can help maneuver baby out.

✦ Prematurity has always been considered a reason for a controlled and monitored bed birth. Some doctors who have experienced the great results of waterbirth for babies born from 36 weeks gestation on, are now questioning whether waterbirth might be good for some babies who are less than 36 weeks gestation. But with the advances in waterproof fetal monitoring there are fewer reasons to require a woman to leave the pool, especially if her baby is tolerating the labor well. A few cases of waterbirth for 33-, 34- and 35-week-old babies have been reported.

Once a woman has experienced a waterbirth she will more than likely want to repeat the experience. To that end, Waterbirth International gets some pretty interesting referral requests from women all over the world. If circumstances have changed and the mother is no longer living in a place where waterbirth facilities or practitioners are readily available, she will go to almost any length to recreate the opportunity to give birth in water. A research project that Waterbirth International has been conducting is a survey of women who have given birth in water. On the survey form is a questions that states, "Would you consider giving birth again in water?" With over 1500 surveys collected, there has only been one woman that answered no to that question. On her particular survey she emphatically stated NO in bold print with two exclamation points and then drew an arrow down to the bottom of the page where in very small print she wrote, "This is number seven; I'm done!"

It is hard to think of another method of childbirth that receives such praise from women and practitioners alike. Dr. Lisa Stolper is an obstetrician practicing in the quaint New England town of Keene, New Hampshire. She began offering waterbirth to her clients at Cheshire Medical Center in October of 1998. One year later she reported an overall waterbirth rate of 37 percent for vaginal births and 33 percent for all births, including cesarean sections. Her hospital has purchased just one portable jetted birth pool, but they use it to labor almost 50 percent of their clients. They are now considering installing permanent pools to make them available for more women. Her comment about her job as an obstetrician was, "Waterbirth just makes my job so much easier."

Why aren't more hospitals in the U.S. offering waterbirth?

Hospitals in the United States have made incredible advances in the waterbirth movement. Monodnock Community Hospital in Peterborough, New Hampshire, was the first hospital in the country to embrace waterbirth and install a permanent birth pool, imported from England. They still offer this option to women and can now look back on almost ten years of great outcomes and lots of satisfied families. The rest of the country has taken some time and there are certain areas of the country that are making greater strides than others. In almost all cases where there are successful waterbirth programs going, they have been started by Certified Nurse Midwives. Midwives are more open to exploring the issue with their clients and doing the research necessary to get protocols accepted in hospitals. Some midwives have even purchased portable birth pool equipment with their own funds in hopes that it would pay for itself by generating more business. In most instances that investment has paid off.

The whole U.S. movement is at least five years behind the European movement in acceptance in hospital environments, but home birth midwives in the U.S. have been offering waterbirth longer than most of their European counterparts.[26] The UK has had the benefit of government-sponsored research and data reporting as well as the Cumberlege Report.[27] The House of Commons Health Committee recommended that all hospitals should provide women with the option of a birthing pool. The underlying philosophy of the "Changing Childbirth" report recognized that women have the right to choose how and where they wish to give birth. In a 1994 statement, the UKCC (United Kingdom Creditation Council) stated, "...waterbirth is preferred by some women as their chosen method for delivery of babies. Waterbirth should therefore be viewed as an alternate method of care and management in labour and one which falls within the midwife's sphere of practice."[28]

The states that have made the most progress for hospital waterbirth are New York, Maine, New Hampshire, Illinois, Ohio, North Carolina, and Massachusetts. Obviously, the East Coast is changing faster than the West Coast. It is surprising to some people when they find out that the whole state of California only has a handful of hospitals that provide waterbirth services. More than two-thirds of the birth centers in the U.S. offer waterbirth as an available option.

Mothers who call Waterbirth International wanting advice on how to get their particular hospital to allow them to have a waterbirth are advised that it takes three ingredients to make policy changes within a hospital setting:

1. a motivated mother,

2. an open and supportive practitioner, and

3. a compassionate nurse manager or perinatal coordinator who is willing to take on the training of staff and the creation of new policy.

Waterbirth International will supply the necessary research studies, the sample protocols, the pool kits, the videos, and the experience to help couples get policy changed, but without these first three components, some hospitals will continue to deny the request.

Time is the other factor. The more advance notice a hospital is given, the better chances there are for change.

The final key to change is education. There are so many areas of waterbirth to explore. Waterbirth is more a philosophy of non-intervention than a method or way to give birth. Waterbirth combines psychology, physiology, technology, humanity, and science. Waterbirth is ancient, and yet new at the same time. Waterbirth embodies a spiritual aspect of birth that is hard to express. Cynthia, who gave birth in water, said it better: "The water made me so completely connected to my body and my baby. The water held me and cradled me so that I could surrender more completely to this amazing and wonderful grace that was happening to me. This is the way that God intended childbirth to be."

9

Birth Plans

✦

Your Declaration of Desires

"It's not easy being a mother. If it were easy, fathers would do it."
  —Erma Bombeck

Your birth plan is your Declaration of Desires, your own personal Birthing Bible, your hospital's Medical Marching Orders, and your Detailed Decree of Do's and Don'ts. It's everything you want to see happen during your entire hospital stay, set in stone.

But within reason.

It should also be very short, very sweet, and very fair. It ought to be considerate, concise, and clear. Its purpose is to list your birthing goals, but be written with everyone in mind.

Composing the birth plan is your newly hired birth professional's first opportunity to be helpful. To start with, she's familiar with the hospitals in your area. If you live in a large city, she's probably been to them, and if you live in a small town, the hospital is familiar territory. She'll know what's routine and what's not, what's offered and what isn't, and how each hospital manages its labor, the birth, pain, and baby care. So, depending on which hospital you choose to use, your birthing professional can tell you what must be made clear in your birth plan and what doesn't have to be mentioned.

I strongly advise that you visit the hospital where you'll be having your baby to see if they have a birth plan form that specifies options they already agree to. Talk to other parents who have had their babies in the hospital you've chosen. Your obstetrician will know of couples who have given birth there, and will have names of some moms who have consented to be reached by phone.

A well thought out birth plan is the perfect means to share your expectations with your doctor so that both of you are on the same page. Go over everything with him in as much detail as necessary, and make sure he understands that this is what you want, that he's comfortable with it, and that he agrees fully with each point. Then *have him sign it*—not because you don't trust him, but because once it's signed it becomes a doctor's order. If no emergencies arise, the hospital staff must follow doctor's orders. This is very important. As a nurse, I know that some instructions written by patients—and not signed by a doctor—aren't binding, so they get placed in the back of the chart and are generally not honored.

The hospital staff also likes to know that you're coming into the hospital well informed and well educated. It makes their job easier when they don't have to explain everything they're doing to you. They'll appreciate not having to guess what you want. If, for example, your birth plan says you want to be up as much as possible, they'll encourage you to get out of bed when they see you've been there too long. If you want only intermittent monitoring of your baby, they'll not just strap the fetal monitor on your tummy and walk off, leaving you attached to a machine. Knowing your desires helps the nursing staff when they're busy. And at change of shift, the off-shift nurse can easily show the oncoming nurse your birth plan, eliminating the need to try to explain all that you want for your birth.

When everything is agreed upon, you can enter the birthing process with confidence. Your doctor understands what's important to you, the hospital staff has their orders, and your birthing professional will be there to make sure the plan is followed every step of the way. You'll be able to put all details out of your mind and focus on what you're there for in the first place.

What is a Birth Plan? There are all kinds of birth plans and lots of ways to put them together. Following are some of the more popular requests I've seen in my practice, as well as pointers I've received from birth attendants across the United States and Canada. I've sorted them under various headings to give you an idea about what you can ask for throughout the labor, birth, and postpartum stages of a normal vaginal birth and what you can ask for should you have a cesarean.

Who Should Have Copies of Your Birth Plan?

+ Your Caregiver
  One for your office chart
  One to send with your records to the birthing site
+ Your Support People
+ The Birthing Site
  One to give to the admitting staff
  One to keep in your birthing room
+ Your Labor Coach
+ You (duh)

The following examples present typical birth plan requests; each one is accompanied by an explanation. But please keep in mind that this is only a set of examples. Your plan will, *and should*, be different.

While in Labor

I'd like no internal fetal monitoring unless absolutely necessary. I'd like to have external monitoring kept to a minimum throughout my labor.

Continuous electronic fetal monitoring may restrict you to the room or even to the bed. This gives you very little chance to walk around and allow gravity to help your baby descend so that the pressure of her head can help dilate your cervix. Lying in bed too long also can cause the baby to lie on her umbilical cord, which can decrease oxygen supply and, in turn, decrease her heart rate. Monitoring has changed in some hospitals; a telemetry-type system now allows you to leave the room and walk around. Still, if you're in early labor and progressing at a steady pace, continuous monitoring isn't necessary.

> Electronic fetal monitoring increased dramatically during the '80s, and disproportionately so for low-risk women, raising questions about the effectiveness of monitoring for improving pregnancy outcomes.[1]

I'd like to use a bathtub while my membranes are still intact and a shower after they've ruptured.

Lying in a tub—after labor is well established—is relaxing and comforting. And hot showers are wonderful, especially when you're feeling most of your discomfort in your back, which is more commonly referred to as back labor. But be aware that getting into a bathtub in early labor can relax the uterus too much and cause contractions to slow down.

Studies have shown that infection rates don't increase when membranes are no longer intact, so some hospitals now allow women to use bathtubs even after their membranes have ruptured.

I don't want to be offered pain medication or an epidural unless an emergency arises and other options have already been tried.

When you're offered pain medication or an epidural your whole thought process starts to change. Once proposed, the idea tends to stick in the back of your mind. When I was attending homebirths my moms never asked for pain medication or wished they had the option, but if they had to go into the hospital, drugs were usually their first request. When I asked one mom what changed her mind, she said that at home she knew she didn't have the choice, but in the hospital all she had to do was bring it up. I asked her if the pain was worse in the hospital and she said no, it was just that the option was available. So if you want a natural childbirth you'll have a much better chance of success if everyone just keeps quiet about pain medications.

I'd like no restrictions on food or drink intake.

Restriction of food and fluids while in labor can cause dehydration and exhaustion. If you become too dehydrated, an IV must be started to replenish the nourishment you'd have been getting from food and drink in the first place. Take some light food with you to the hospital. Flavored gelatins, puddings, or even fruits are easy to bring and easy to digest. You should drink at least eight ounces of water or fruit juice every hour or two to keep your strength up and to keep you urinating. You should go to the bathroom every hour or two to keep your bladder empty—a full bladder will slow the descent of your baby.

> Recent studies on oral hydration and food intake suggest that women who are allowed to eat and drink to comfort in labor have shorter labor (by an average of 90 minutes), less need for augmentation with Pitocin, require fewer pain medications, and their babies had higher Apgar scores than of those in the control group.[2]

Upon admission, I don't want a routine IV or heplock started unless there's an emergency. IV pain management can be given intravenously by syringe to the hand.

There's no need for a routine IV when you're admitted to the hospital. Once an IV is started, the staff has easy access for other interventions, setting a precedent for further meddling. If you need an IV later it can be started later—it takes only a few minutes. A heplock (an IV access without the fluids infusing) can become very irritating when you're in labor, and chances are that if you're having your baby naturally you won't need it anyway. If pain medication becomes a must, it can be quickly administered with a short needle in a vein in your hand.

Unless discussed beforehand, I don't want my labor and birth to be placed on a time limit. Examples: dilating one centimeter per hour, or birthing my baby X hours after rupture of membranes.

Very often hospital policy dictates that moms must dilate at least one centimeter per hour. Obviously, this average rate of dilation doesn't apply to all births. If the infant's heart rate shows that he's tolerating the labor and your contractions are steady and strong, intervention is simply not necessary. Basing labor's progress on the rate of dilation sets up a success/failure scenario: if your physician decides your labor isn't progressing fast enough to meet their standards, they may decide to start an IV solution of Pitocin to accelerate your contractions. Your birthing professional will help enforce your desire not to be placed on a time schedule because she can help monitor your laboring process and relay the information to your nurse.

I'd like internal vaginal exams kept to a minimum. I prefer to have the exam at my request if I have a desire to push or if my contractions change significantly.

A vaginal exam is usually done when you're admitted to see how far your labor has progressed. After that, vaginal exams should be kept to a minimum because they open the door to infection, especially if your membranes aren't intact. Frequent exams can also cause unnecessary distress if you're not progressing rapidly. And the staff can use the exams to justify putting you on a time schedule. The initial exam is the only time you should be examined until you're ready to push.

I don't want my membranes to be artificially ruptured to augment labor or to accelerate my contractions. But if my labor must be accelerated, I prefer that over Pitocin.

Artificially rupturing your membranes puts you at risk for being placed on a time schedule. When a woman's membranes are ruptured, the hospital usually requires that you birth your baby within a specified time frame because of the risk of infection. If rupturing your membranes is successful but doesn't hasten labor, your provider will probably want to start Pitocin to speed up your labor, and birth you soon to avoid the risk of infection. One other major risk that could be brought about by artificially rupturing your membranes would be cord prolapse. When membranes are ruptured and the baby's head is high in the birth canal, the cord could slip past his head and out through the cervix. Without the cushion of water between the head and the pelvic structure, the head rapidly engages on the pelvic floor, and if the cord is between the baby's head and the pelvic bones the baby's oxygen will be cut off. If this happens the baby will have to be born by cesarean.

> If a woman feels threatened, or if her surroundings are even slightly unfamiliar, labor may slow or stop. For this reason some mothers choose to remain at home throughout early labor and some active labor.

We'd like the labor room to be as quiet and undisturbed as possible, with lights dimmed and minimal nurse visits.

You'll be able to relax and labor more effectively if your environment is quiet, darkened and undisturbed, and you're surrounded by familiar and friendly faces. I've attended births where for no obvious reason the mother's labor suddenly slowed down and became more painful and uncomfortable. When I stood back and observed the room, I saw an undercurrent of chaos and confusion. After I cleared the room of those who didn't really belong, made the room quiet and dimmed the lights, the mom regained her focus and established a productive labor pattern.

During Your Baby's Birth

If I have an epidural I'd like it shut off or turned way down when I'm about 8 centimeters dilated or when it's one to two hours before the time to push.

Successful pushing is based on how much you feel the desire. Because an epidural is likely to render you numb from the waist down, you won't feel the urge to push unless it's turned off or drastically reduced. Even decreasing the dose will help you feel the urge to push. When you can tell your midwife or doctor that you're having a contraction and feel like pushing, it'll help her encourage you and give you support. Having the epidural shut off will also help you have enough feeling in your legs to position them to help make the passage larger for the baby.

I'd like heat, ice, or oil used instead of a perineal massage, and I want to avoid an episiotomy if possible.

Dr. Una Jean Sayles, in all her wisdom, said that massaging the perineum prior to pushing actually increases blood flow and causes tissues to swell. This in turn causes the perineum to thicken, decreasing the chance of it remaining intact. But when heat, ice, or oil was applied to the perineum, the muscles relaxed and stretched easily. I've also found that when heat or ice is applied to the perineum during the pushing phase, the perineum visibly relaxes and mom knows what she's pushing against to expel her baby. Oil poured over the perineum and baby's head during the birth also helps slide the baby out without tearing the perineum.

I'd like to hold off injecting the perineum with Lidocaine (for numbing) until after the baby is born, even with an episiotomy.

Injecting Lidocaine into the perineum before a tear or episiotomy adds fluid and thickens the tissues, making it harder for the muscles to stretch. If an episiotomy is truly necessary, the best time to do it is when the baby begins to crown and the area is at its thinnest. When the perineum is stretched that tight, cutting usually doesn't hurt. Then after the baby is born Lidocaine can be administered for suturing purposes.

According to a Clinical Commentary in the April 2000 issue of *Obstetrics & Gynecology* and posted on the America College of Obstetricians and Gynecologists web site (acog.org), "Episiotomy should *not* [emphasis mine] be a routine part of labor and delivery." Even so, the authors of the commentary determined that "the procedure is still performed too frequently" (in 1996, it was performed in about 33% of live births) and the results didn't show that episiotomies "decreased incidents of urinary incontinence."

An episiotomy, as defined in the article, is an incision "made into the perineum area between the vagina and the anus" in order to "widen the vaginal opening and help shorten delivery time." It used to be thought that it would "prevent maternal pelvic organ prolapse, urinary incontinence, and lacerations that healed poorly." Doctors also used to think that laboring too long could lead to "trauma, cerebral palsy, and other neurological disorders" in the baby. Based on several studies, both short- and long-term, however, the authors of the commentary, Erica Eason, MDCM, FRCSC, from the Department of Obstetrics and Gynecology at the University of Ottawa, and Perle Feldman, MDCM, FCFP, from the Department of Family Medicine at McGill University in Toronto, say none of that is true.

> An article in *Obstetrics and Gynecology*[3], August 2000, said that routine episiotomy is no longer advisable. Unfortunately, the practice continues. A woman giving birth vaginally in America today has at least a 40 percent chance of receiving an episiotomy. A research review by the World Health Organization, however, indicates that evidence only supports a 5- to 20-percent rate.

The authors assessed many short- and long-term studies that compared "women who delivered with an episiotomy to those who didn't," and studies on the "development of infants delivered after an extended second stage of labor compared with those delivered after an episiotomy." "No significant differences in infant outcome" were found. Indeed, for some conditions of the mother, "women without episiotomies fared as well or better than women who received episiotomies."

When long-term studies that followed children until age seven and "examined their IQ and motor deficits" were checked, the authors found "no correlation between poor neurological outcomes and length of labor."

Other studies showed that mothers "with intact perineums or those who delivered via cesarean," when compared with women with episiotomies, had stronger "pelvic floors and were therefore less likely to end up with a worse prolapse." Further, the studies revealed "no differences in incidence of urinary incontinence" between the groups. In addition, those mothers that hadn't had an episiotomy "experienced less blood loss, less risk of infection, and less perineal pain after delivery."

I'd like other choices of pushing positions besides the standard supine position with leg stirrups.

"Because the uterus is titling upward when you are lying on your back, pushing your baby out in [the lithotomy] position is like having a bowel movement while standing on your head," Dr. Una Jean Sayles, a family practice physician with whom I did over 200 births in Canada (and who also helped

> The word "obstetrician" comes from Latin, and it means "to stand before."

me birth my own children at home), once said. Pushing while squatting with the help of a squat bar, while on your hands and knees, or while lying on your side helps the birth of your baby because you're not fighting gravity. Even just sitting up a bit or having your partner sit behind you cradling you and offering support will allow gravity to help bring your baby out. Ask your midwife or doctor what other birthing positions she has seen used, and ask other moms and birth professionals what works best for them.

If the need arises, I prefer vacuum extraction rather than forceps.

Vacuum extraction causes fewer complications to the baby than forceps births. Fortunately, this is becoming common knowledge. According to the February 1999 Cochrane Review of vacuum extraction versus forceps for assisted vaginal births, the use of vacuum extractors rather than forceps for assisted births appeared to reduce maternal morbidity in the ten trials that were examined. The review also noted that with the use of vacuum extraction there was a reduction in cephalhematoma (a collection of blood under the scalp) and retinal hemorrhages.

I'd like my partner to cut the cord after it has stopped pulsating, and I want my baby placed on my chest immediately. I also want all routine medications for my baby delayed for at least two hours to give us time to nurse and bond.

If there were no complications and baby is okay, then routine procedures such as eye drops, vitamin K, and so forth can be tended to later. The newborn exam can actually be done while you're holding your baby. If your child is chilled, rather than use warming lights the baby can be placed skin-to-skin with you, with both of you wrapped in blankets. Warming lights take longer, and they expose the baby to open spaces, which they really, really hate because they're used to the cozy close quarters of the womb.

I'd like to expel the placenta completely unassisted— no Pitocin, uterine massage, or cord traction.

Physicians are trained to have the placenta expelled within five minutes after birth. They're taught to tug on the cord and irritate the uterus until it contracts, or to massage the fundus to stimulate a contraction. I've even seen physicians wrap the cord around hemostats and pull. I've also seen the cord snap off and the poor mother and baby hemorrhage.

If we let nature take its course, the placenta expels naturally in about thirty minutes. After baby is born and placed on your chest, she will take time to adjust to the new environment by checking things out for fifteen or twenty minutes. Then the instinct to suck kicks in, and she'll start to root (search for the breast). When the baby is placed on the breast she immediately latches on, and the sucking will stimulate your body to release oxytocin into your system. This causes the placenta to detach from the uterine wall and the uterus to contract and expel it. Presto. Mother Nature does it again—it just takes a little patience from the doctor.

Newborn Care

I don't want my baby suctioned or deep-suctioned unless absolutely necessary.

Suctioning can cause trauma to the airway if done improperly. If baby is born pink, breathing on his or her own, and has a good cry, then chances are good that he doesn't need routine suctioning at all.

I want to breastfeed as soon as my baby shows signs of interest and not before.

Babies need about fifteen to twenty minutes before their instinct to breastfeed hits. Trying to force him into it before he is ready can cause frustration for both of you. When babies are born and placed on their mom's tummy, they first lie quietly with their eyes closed. After about five minutes they open their eyes, look around, and explore their first sensations in the big outside world. They listen to sounds, feel the temperature of the room, and smell their mommy. After about twenty minutes they feel an urge to suck and start rooting on their mother's chest. When they're brought to the nipple they eagerly latch on and successfully have their first meal. When babies learn to breastfeed this way, with patience and on their own time, they continue to be good breastfeeders with fewer complications.

I don't want my baby offered a bottle or a pacifier at any time. If my baby cries in the nursery I want him brought to me.

Offering a baby a bottle or pacifier will only confuse them and make breastfeeding more difficult to establish. Getting nourishment from a bottle is much easier for babies—all they have to do is slightly push the rubber nipple against the roof of their mouth with their tongue and milk will flow. With a breast, babies have to suck much harder and wait until the milk lets down before it even gets to them. Quite frankly, they are lazy little darlings, and they'll always take the easy way out. So please, for the first two weeks at least, refrain from offering a pacifier or bottle. Supplements, if necessary, can be given with a medicine cup and, surprisingly, a baby will actually sip from it.

I'd like my partner, myself, or my birth professional to be present during all newborn procedures. I'd also like to have all procedures explained to us before they are done.

These requests are not out of line and are well within your rights. Some procedures are done in the nursery, not in the mom's room. If mom is too sick or sore to go with the baby, then she can appoint someone else to go each time. If no one is there to accompany the baby and if it isn't an emergency, then the procedure can be done later.

Cesarean Section Plan

If I need to have a cesarean section I want my husband and/or my birth professional present in the operating room at all times.

Operating rooms are not exactly famous for their calming effects. If you need a cesarean, having someone familiar with you will help ease your anxieties. The person who is with you can sit at your head and talk to you because most C-sections are done with spinal anesthesia while the mom is awake.

If time allows we'd like to discuss anesthesia options. This applies to anesthesia for C-section as well as regular vaginal birth.

Two people are involved when you're considering anesthesia: you and your baby. The perfect anesthetic will provide pain relief and allow you to push when you're ready and have a baby who isn't too sleepy. Sedation by means of IV narcotics is generally used during labor, and I've found that they only make a mom sleepy and don't help relieve painful contractions. In fact, they make mom so sleepy during the beginning of a contraction that when she wakes from the discomfort of it she's already at the peak and most painful part. Not being able to start your labor breathing at the very beginning of the contraction can make it unbearable and you'll not be able to establish a nice rhythm.

An epidural is a local anesthetic that's delivered in the back just outside of the spinal cord. It provides a continuous infusion of narcotic and renders the mom numb from the waist down. The chapter on medications discusses this technique more fully. A C-section can be done while a mom is using an epidural, or a general anesthesia can be used to put the mom completely to sleep. Be sure to ask questions: Will I remember everything? Will it affect my baby? Will I be able to breastfeed?

> Neither husbands, nor lovers, nor prospective grandparents, nor prospective adoptive parents, nor adoption agencies have a right to consent to, or interfere in, the medical care of the pregnant woman.[4]

I'd like my baby to stay with my husband or birthing professional until I am ready to join them.

After you see your baby in the operating room and the baby is stable, she can follow your partner to your postpartum room and not go to the nursery. This will also give your partner a special time to bond with the baby before you return to the room.

I'd like to have my baby with me at all times and not taken to the nursery unless I ask.

After a C-section the mother is usually encouraged to have her baby put in the nursery some of the time to allow her to rest. During the first twenty-four hours the baby is at risk for aspirating fluids he has not expelled from his lungs. After a C-section you can't jump out of bed if your baby is choking, so it's a good idea to have someone in your room with you and your baby, especially while you're sleeping.

Wrap up

Well that's it. Use these ideas as food for thought, discuss them with your husband and birthing professional, and draft your own birth plan. Remember to keep it straightforward, clear and, above all, short and sweet. I'm not encouraging you to use all these ideas—listing too many conditions will seem overly demanding, and your doctor might hesitate to sign it. Or the staff might consider you too difficult and be less willing to work with you. But when you have a well thought out birth plan, clearly written and signed by your doctor, you're golden.

Birth Plan

There are many options to consider. Fill out, circle, or check what's important to you and cross out the ones you couldn't care less about. Have fun, talk to others, and take your time. REMEMBER: *Have your provider sign this contract when you're done.* This makes it "Doctor's Orders" and it can't be ignored. I've seen carefully thought out—but unsigned—birth plans placed in the back of the patient's chart and never used or even looked at again. But ones that are signed by a provider are treated as orders and **have** to be honored. So, one last time, *after you're done with your birth plan have your provider sign and date it.*

Birthing Plan for: _____

Who I'd like with me during labor: _____

Who I'd like to stay for my baby's birth: _____

During My Labor

1. I want to bring all kinds of food and drink:

   _____

   _____

2. Diversions to keep me occupied during labor:

   Music _____

   Videos _____

   Books/magazines _____

   Games/puzzles _____

   Other _____

3. For any discomfort, I'd like:

   ❏ Water therapy, shower, or tub
   ❏ Coaching with breathing and relaxation
   ❏ IV/IM pain relief, Demerol, stadol, morphine
   ❏ Oral pain medications such as Vicodin, Tylenol 3, or Percocet
   ❏ Epidural
   ❏ Other _____

	Yes	No
4. I don't want an IV or heplock unless it is medically necessary.	❏	❏
5. I don't want unnecessary lab work just because it's routine.	❏	❏
6. I don't care if my room is noisy and full of people.	❏	❏
7. I don't want my labor put on a time limit.	❏	❏

8. If my water needs breaking, I would like it to be:

❏ When I'm past 5 centimeters dilated

❏ If I've not progressed for a couple of hours

❏ After my baby's head is well engaged

❏ Other _____

9. I'd like to be vaginally examined:

❏ When I'm admitted

❏ Before any pain meds

❏ When I feel like pushing

❏ When I ask for it

During My Baby's Birth

	Yes	No
1. If I have an epidural I want it shut off after I am ____ cm dilated or ____ hours before I'm expected to have my baby.	❏	❏
2. If I have an epidural and my labor stops I don't want Pitocin.	❏	❏
3. While I'm pushing I'd like ❏ heat ❏ oil ❏ other _____ applied to my perineum.	❏	❏
4. I don't want an episiotomy before my baby is born. I'd rather have a slow birth and take my chances.	❏	❏
5. I don't want Lidocaine injected into my perineum for suturing after my baby is born.	❏	❏
6. I don't want Lidocaine injected into my perineum if I tear or need an episiotomy.	❏	❏

7. I'd like to try alternate positions for pushing:

❏ Squatting

❏ Squatting Bar

❏ Hands and Knees

❏ Side Lying

❏ Other _____

8. If my baby needs assistance being born I want vacuum extraction rather than forceps.	❏	❏
9. I care if the cord stops pulsating before it's cut.	❏	❏
10. I care if the physician uses Pitocin to expel my placenta.	❏	❏

After I Have My Baby

	Yes	No

1. I want to breastfeed my baby, and I want my baby at my breast within _____ minutes after birth.   ❏   ❏

2. I want my baby offered a bottle or pacifier.   ❏   ❏

3. I want all of my baby's procedures done in my room and my baby kept with me at all times.   ❏   ❏

4. If I cannot go myself, I want my baby accompanied by my husband or birth partner during any procedures.   ❏   ❏

5. If my baby and I are fine, I'd like to be released _____ hours after my baby is born.   ❏   ❏

Cesarean Section Considerations

1. I want my husband and/or birth professional with me during the operation.   ❏   ❏

2. I want to discuss anesthetic options with my anesthesiologist.   ❏   ❏

3. I want my baby returned to my room (rather than the nursery) with my husband or birth professional while I'm in recovery.   ❏   ❏

4. I don't want my baby taken to the nursery while I sleep (I will provide someone for care).   ❏   ❏

10
Breastfeeding

✦

Congratulations, You've Got Milk!

"Now, as always, the most automated appliance in a household is the mother."
—Beverly Jones

lthough breastfeeding is a natural process and gazillions of moms have successfully done it, for some it's just not that easy. But that doesn't mean it's impossible. My mother didn't breastfeed me, and neither did she tell me what to expect or how to prepare for it. But I was lucky—I had fantastic help and support from my friend and midwifery partner and successfully nursed each of my daughters for two years. I doubt I could have pulled it off without Sandy's help and guidance.

Most likely the doula partner you choose will have read a lot about breastfeeding and may also be experienced at it. She can give you plenty of advice, both before the birth and after you have your baby. Most birth doulas are available for postpartum care, so she can come to your home after your baby is born and support your efforts to breastfeed as well as relieve you of daily chores and responsibilities.

I have always loved teaching breastfeeding skills to new moms. I have worked with moms who have had trouble getting started and showed them ways they can be successful at breastfeeding. That's what this chapter is all about, so let's get started!

Breastfeeding and Intelligence.
Increasing duration of breastfeeding is associated with consistent and statistically significant:

✦ increase in intelligence quotients of 5 points or more at 8 years old and as adults

✦ higher reading, mathematics, and overall scholastic ability at 10–13 years old

✦ higher levels in school-leaving examinations

— Horwood *et al*, *Pediatrics*, 1998, 101(1):e9

Breastfed babies have fewer incidences of:

+ ear infections
+ allergies
+ meningitis
+ pneumonia
+ vomiting
+ diarrhea
+ sudden infant death syndrome (SIDS)

It is recommended that mothers breastfeed for one year or longer because breast milk:

+ is easier for babies to digest
+ comes ready to use
+ is free

Besides, breastfeeding is good for moms as well because it:

+ burns calories and helps mom reduce her pregnancy weight
+ reduces the risk of ovarian and breast cancer
+ builds bone strength
+ delays the return of menses, and therefore provides a degree of birth control. (Cautionary note: Don't rely on it as your only way to prevent pregnancy.)
+ helps the uterus return to its normal size.

What's so good about breastfeeding your baby?

Human milk is designed for human babies, just as dog's milk is designed for puppies and cat's milk for kittens. Every species creates exactly what their young ones need for nourishment in order to thrive. So your milk provides all the protein, fat, sugar, and vitamins your baby needs to stay healthy as well as protective substances to protect her from diseases and infections.

How do I get help with breastfeeding?

The first, second, and third things to do are research, research, and research. Before you have your baby, take time to read, watch videos, and learn all you can about breastfeeding. Some hospitals offer classes, and organizations such as La Leche League International offer tons of information. Ask your midwife, obstetrician, pediatrician, or doula for local phone numbers of support groups and classes. Planned Parenthood offers information too, as do prenatal caregivers. Your midwife's or doctor's staff can help you line up a breastfeeding advocate in your area, and many hospitals are now employing lactation consultants who can direct you to breastfeeding instructors and advocates.

What is colostrum?

As soon as you become pregnant, your body starts to prepare for breastfeeding. At about the fourth or fifth month you're already capable of producing pre-milk, or colostrum, which is thick and yellowish, and full of white blood cells and infection-fighting proteins that your baby needs because his immune system isn't fully matured. When new germs enter your body, you develop antibodies to destroy them. These antibodies are transferred to your baby through your colostrum.

The baby gets colostrum for two to three days after the birth before your mature milk comes in. If you cannot breastfeed, at least pump for the first three days to provide your baby with the antibodies he needs to stay healthy.

What is mature milk?

By the third or fourth day of active breastfeeding, your mature milk will come in. The colostrum you produced in the beginning is replaced with what looks more like skim milk. The feel of your breasts will change too—they'll go from feeling soft to feeling firm, with a sensation of fullness. The fullness may cause tenderness and be uncomfortable. You may want to wear a support bra during this time and while breastfeeding.

What hormones are responsible for producing milk?

When you breastfeed, your body produces prolactin, a hormone that stimulates the breasts to make milk. Your baby's sucking prompts nerve sensors in your nipples to send messages to your pituitary gland to secrete prolactin. (Prolactin is also called the mothering hormone because it is thought to form the chemical basis for "mother's intuition.")

With continued sucking these same nerve sensors stimulate and release another hormone called oxytocin. This causes the milk glands to contract, squeezing a large supply of richer milk with extra fat into the ducts and sinuses and eventually to the nipples for your hungry baby. Oxytocin also helps contract your uterus every time you breastfeed. The contractions help return it to its pre-pregnant state and help control bleeding in the first few days. The cramping you feel as you breastfeed will last only about one week, and using the breathing and relaxation techniques you learned for labor will help ease the discomfort.

There is an interesting article by Kayley Fjording on *bambi-bangkok.org/magazine/2000/b_jun00.htm*. Titled "Hormone of love," in it she tells us that "Oxytocin is known as the 'hormone of love'." She says it is "responsible for men's protective behavior, and women's caring and nurturing actions," and that it has "a vital role in orgasm, labor, and breastfeeding." She indicates that fluctuations in the levels of oxytocin provide "the rhythm of the contractions, or opening of the cervix," and that "whatever will provide the right climate for good lovemaking" also makes for "good labor," because "rising oxytocin levels are needed for each." Adrenaline, which is produced "when you feel frightened or anxious," needs to be controlled because it "impedes the production of oxytocin."

Should I do anything to prepare my breasts for feeding?

Not much. Just be sure that you buy properly fitting bras and use only warm water when washing your breasts. Soap and lotions aren't necessary and may irritate the nipples.

What about inverted nipples?

If you have inverted nipples, your baby may have trouble grasping the areola (the dark-colored area surrounding the nipple) properly to get milk. Using a breast pump a few minutes before you actually put the baby to breast will draw the nipples out. You can either use a hand pump or rent an electric one. The hospital will probably give you a shield to place over your nipple that gives your baby something to grasp when he sucks. It also helps pull your nipple out. Be sure to consult the lactation consultant before you go home from the hospital, or if you're planning a homebirth, check with one before your due date. She'll be able to give you some tips about how to successfully nurse your baby.

When should I first feed my baby?

It's best to start breastfeeding within an hour after having your baby. Babies have natural instincts for survival that must be acted upon within a certain time after they're born; babies who don't go to the breast soon actually lose their instinct to nurse and must relearn the process. So babies who are placed to the breast and encouraged to nurse right away are usually more successful than those who are separated from mom.

Time and time again I have witnessed this most amazing natural instinct. If you allow your baby to choose his own time to latch on, you'll not only have a successful first attempt but your placenta will more easily expel. Immediately after your baby is born he should be placed on your chest, skin-to-skin. About five minutes later your baby will look around and check out his new environment. An average of twenty minutes later he'll start rooting, tapping his mouth on your chest looking for his first meal. If you present your nipple at that instant he'll usually clamp on and start feeding right away. It's one of the most emotional moments you'll ever experience.

What about positions?

There are several positions for breastfeeding. I'll describe some here, but you should discuss all the options with your doula. She'll help you choose the one that's best for you and your baby.

Babies are very sensitive to texture. Everything is new to them, and nothing feels better to them than their mommy. Before you start nursing your baby, have the room very warm and strip all baby's clothes off except for a diaper. You can put a blanket around her after she begins nursing. Place your nearly-naked baby to your breast on her side so that your baby's stomach is touching your stomach. Like us, a baby cannot suck and swallow if her head is turned, so be sure her mouth is aligned with her trunk. Baby can see clearly to about nine inches away—about the distance from your face to your nipple. She can see pretty clearly whatever eye contact you make with her while nursing.

If you've had a vaginal birth, you have several position options. The traditional cradle position is the most popular. Sit up, put a pillow or two on your lap, and place your naked baby, on his side, stomach-to-stomach with you. If you start with the left breast, support his body and head with your right arm wrapped behind his body, and place your hand on the back of his neck and head. With your left hand, elbow out, grasp your fingers around your left breast with fingers away from the areola (the brown area around your nipple) and pull slightly back so the nipple stands out. Gently guide your baby's head with your right hand to your breast and tap his mouth on your nipple until he opens it wide enough to take the entire nipple and some of the areola. Then push his mouth over the nipple and gently hold it there. He will start licking and experimenting with sucking. Keep still and try not to distract him with movement or noise. Eventually he will clamp on and start sucking. If he gets upset or starts crying and pulling back, stop and soothe him, staying calm and quiet. When he has settled down, try again. He will eventually catch on to what you are doing and have his meal.

I like the football hold, and my moms have usually had good luck with it. Sit up and place pillows beside you (the left side, in this example). This time hold your baby as you would a football, tucking her under your arm, again on her side with her stomach and chest touching your side. She should be wrapped around your side with her mouth at nipple height. Your left arm is wrapped around her body with your left hand holding the back of her neck and head. With your right hand, grasp your breast as you did before, pulling back slightly to make your nipple stick out. Tease her with the tapping as before; when her mouth opens wide place her mouth over the nipple and areola. Let her play with it until she starts sucking. Again, it may take patience and several attempts. If you give her time and don't give in to using a bottle or pacifier, she will learn this is her means of nutrition, and soon she will be a successful breastfeeder.

If you have had a cesarean birth, the cradle hold may be too painful because baby is placed over the incision. I always encourage C-section moms to try the football hold first. Always position lots of pillows around you and under the baby when you breastfeed; this will help with incisional pain—remember, you've just had major abdominal surgery.

The side-lying position is another option. It uses the same principle as the cradle and football holds, but mom is lying on her side, stomach to stomach with the baby. Wrap your arm around your baby so you can guide your baby's head to the nipple. This takes a little practice and is difficult to do in the hospital because the beds are way too narrow. It will definitely be easier to do at home and very convenient for night feedings. Have your partner help you change position, because turning with a cesarean incision is painful for the first couple of days.

Explain what proper latching-on means.

A correctly latched-on baby will:
✦ cause better milk flow,
✦ help prevent overly full breasts,
✦ keep baby satisfied,
✦ prevent sore nipples, and
✦ stimulate a good milk supply.

An improperly latched-on baby can cause very sore and cracked nipples, so placing your baby to your breast properly is very important. While you're initially tapping his mouth to your nipple, be sure he opens very wide before pressing him to your nipple. Once he is nursing, make sure that most of the areola is drawn into his mouth. A baby's lips and gums should be around the areola, with lips visible. Be sure your fingers are well out of the way of your baby's grasp of the nipple. If you feel pain from baby's sucking or hear smacking noises, then he is not latched on properly, and you will end up with very sore nipples. Pull him off and try again.

What about occasionally using bottles?

While you and your baby are learning to breastfeed, you should never give your baby supplements unless it is medically necessary. Offering your baby a bottle or even a pacifier in the beginning will only confuse her. The first two weeks of breastfeeding are the most crucial; during this time you and your baby will learn to become the perfect nursing couple. Babies are lazy little creatures; if they're given the choice between sucking hard on the breast or taking in the relatively easy flow from a bottle, guess which she'll choose.

What about giving baby breast milk from a bottle?

I know, when you're tired or heading out for the night, it sounds like a good idea to have someone feed your baby from a bottle. But this may confuse your baby about where he's getting his milk from, and may even start the weaning process. If daddy, grandma or a sibling is feeling left out and wants to be involved in the care of the new baby, they can choose to be the one who goes to the baby when he is hungry, change his diaper and give him to mommy to feed. Then, when mommy is done breastfeeding, they can burp baby and rock him back to sleep. Not only will they be having special time with baby, they will be helping mommy get the rest she needs.

What does "milk let-down" mean?

In order for your baby to draw milk from your breast, the "let-down" reflex must occur. This means milk is ejected from the milk glands to the milk sinuses. Let-down can be felt in many different ways. Many women feel a light tingling in the upper breasts, whereas others experience a slightly painful tingling. Milk may occasionally leak from your breast when you hear a baby crying or when you start nursing on the opposite side. If the thought of this concerns you, you can use nursing pads or cover your breasts lightly with squares of clean cloth. Be sure the pads aren't plastic-lined; air should be allowed to circulate and keep your breasts dry so your nipples stay healthy.

These discomforts and inconveniences will eventually clear up when your body adjusts to its new role. In the meantime, here are some things you can do to ease the let-down process:

+ Correctly position your baby so he's properly latched onto the breast.

+ Get comfortable in an easy chair or on the bed, with pillows surrounding you.

+ Listen to your favorite music and sip a soothing beverage such as tea or juice while you nurse.

+ Choose a quiet place to nurse.

+ Don't smoke, drink alcohol, or use illegal drugs—they can severely interfere with the let-down reflex.

+ Wear comfortable, well-fitting bras and clothing that can be easily opened.

+ While you're nursing your baby, a calm review of what your body is doing can help the milk ducts relax and release milk.

What special care do my breasts need during breastfeeding?

Basically, dry them after you breastfeed. Pat them dry with a clean cloth, or let them air dry before you put on your bra.

Avoid soap. It can cause dryness and cracking and remove natural oils that protect your nipples. If they become sore or cracked, try applying either expressed breast milk or any lanolin cream for breastfeeding moms, which promotes healing by stimulating the production of natural tissue moisture.

How frequently should I breastfeed my baby?

Breastfed babies eat more frequently than formula-fed babies. Formula's greater density is harder to digest than breast milk and makes baby feel full longer. So expect your breastfed baby to eat eight to twelve times a day or more. During the first three to four weeks your baby will probably nurse every couple of hours, but by the end of the first month your baby will be taking in enough to probably allow him to sleep at least five hours during the night. But remember, all babies are different; yours may not sleep that long.

If you really want to know when your baby is hungry, feed him only on demand. Throw out the clocks and don't set the timers. Let your baby tell you when he is hungry.

When your baby is hungry she may do several things:

+ start the rooting reflex

+ put her hands to her mouth and make sucking motions

+ cry vigorously

+ nuzzle into your breast

Frequent wakefulness is another problem babies can develop. Usually it simply means they are not getting enough to eat during feedings. Baby may fall asleep after breastfeeding for only five minutes on one side; she then wakes up an hour later, frantic and wanting to nurse again. This pattern doesn't give mom or baby time to rest. When you breastfeed your baby, she should nurse at least 15 to 30 minutes on one side. If she is sleepy, change her diaper, wake her up, and place her on the other breast for another 15 to 30 minutes. This will fill her tummy, empty both breasts, and likely ensure that she will sleep a good three hours between feedings.

> A cautionary note: If during the first month postpartum your baby goes longer than three and a half to four hours before wanting to breastfeed, wake her before she becomes overly hungry. If she goes too long between feedings, she may become frantic, anxious, and hard to calm down. When they get to this point, babies are often unable to successfully latch on to the breast.

What is engorgement?

One of the most uncomfortable and painful things that can happen to breastfeeding moms is engorgement, associated with the sudden increase in milk volume, lymphatic and vascular congestion, and interstitial edema during the two weeks following. The breasts will feel hard and become extremely tender and sore, and the skin will feel tight. The breasts can swell so much that it causes the milk ducts to seal off, and you won't be able to release milk from your breasts. This situation can be prevented by nursing frequently—at least every two to three hours for at least ten to fifteen minutes on each side. Alternate sides each time you start breastfeeding. For example, if you start on the right side for one feeding, start on the left side the next time. The baby sucks hardest the first fifteen minutes, so alternating ensures that you empty your breasts evenly. Wear a good-quality nursing bra, one that doesn't have under-wires or is too tight. Try to sleep on your back to keep your breasts elevated. Also, cold packs to the breasts help with some of the swelling after feedings.

> WHO, UNICEF, and the American Academy of Pediatrics all recommend exclusive (i.e. only) breastfeeding for 6 months, continued breastfeeding for at least 12 months, and longer if mutually desired by infant and mother.

If you become engorged, try these ideas:

✦ Apply heat to your breasts before you begin breastfeeding to help the milk ducts relax and release milk. Run a disposable diaper (because it holds the water in the diaper and won't drip out) under hot water, then place it to your breasts. Be sure the water is not so hot it scalds you.

✦ Sometimes ice will reduce swelling. Between feedings, try putting bags of frozen peas or corn in your bra.

✦ Before you breastfeed, express some milk manually or with an electric pump placed on minimum, then gradually increasing pressure. Sometimes it helps to pump after you breastfeed so all the milk is drained from your breasts.

✦ Try different breastfeeding positions—football hold, cradle hold, sitting, or lying down. This allows baby to latch on differently and drain different milk ducts.

✦ Gently massage your breasts, starting under the arm and working toward the nipple. This helps reduce soreness and ease milk flow.

✦ Consult your physician first if you think you need pain medication.

Don't stop breastfeeding because you are engorged. It's only a temporary condition! The more you empty your breasts the more quickly the condition will subside. In fact, frequent breastfeeding helps keep the milk in your breasts emptied, prevents you from being overly full, and prevents engorgement.

Cabbage leaf compress: This is an old-fashioned remedy that sounds a little odd, but I've seen it work successfully many times. Cut the hard part off several cabbage leaves and refrigerate the leaves until they are good and cold. Then place the leaves on your engorged breast, but not on the nipple, and leave them place for about twenty minutes. The breasts should soften; in some incidences I've even seen milk drip from the nipple. When your breasts feel soft, or if you start dripping milk, put baby to breast or use a pump to drain some of the milk. Repeat this routine a couple of times between feedings. Sipping some Mothers Milk™ herbal tea can do wonders to help this remedy along. Take heart—engorgement usually lasts for only about one to two days if you actively work at resolving it.

How do I express milk?

You can express milk from your breasts for later use either manually or with an electric pump. An electric breast pump has much better sucking and drawing capabilities than a manual pump, but is more costly and less portable.

To express milk manually:

1. Make sure your hands and the equipment are clean.

2. Put a clean container under your breast.

3. Massage each breast gently, working toward the nipple. You may also want to apply heat with a cloth diaper moistened with hot water.

4. Place thumb and forefinger on the top and bottom of the nipple.

5. Press the nipple back toward your chest, then gently pinch and release the areola between your thumb and forefinger in a rhythmic motion until the milk flows or squirts out.

6. Occasionally reposition your thumb and forefinger around the nipple to stimulate all the ducts.

Store the captured milk in a clean, covered container in the refrigerator or freezer for later feedings (see the next section).

Electric pumps usually include two plastic bottles, each with an attachment (cone) that fits over the nipples. Plastic tubing attaches the cones to a machine/pump that creates a vacuum when it is attached to the nipples. The pump has three settings, or sucking strengths—minimum to maximum. Place the cones on your nipples and start the machine on the "minimum" setting. The suction action will gently start drawing your nipples into the cones and extract milk from your breasts; it's done in waves to simulate the sucking of a baby. Use the machine for about fifteen minutes. When you feel comfortable during this time you can increase the strength to maximum. Refrigerate or freeze your milk in clean, covered containers.

Talk to your practitioner about the various types of electric breast pumps and where you can buy or rent one. She will also be able to show you how to operate and clean it.

How do I store breast milk properly?

+ Store milk in sterile screw-cap bottles, glass, any freezer container that is specifically made for freezing foods, or heavy-grade nursery bags that are freezer-safe. An example is the one made by Playtex, initially used as inserts for baby bottles. Sealed milk can be safely stored in the refrigerator for 72 hours, in the freezer part of a one-door refrigerator for two weeks, in a conventional two-door refrigerator/freezer for two to three months, and in a zero-degree freezer for up to six months.

+ Freeze two to four ounces per container.

+ Do not add fresh milk to already-frozen milk.

+ Don't use a microwave to thaw or heat milk. It doesn't heat evenly and may burn the baby's mouth. The best way to heat milk is to place the container in a larger container of hot water.

+ Thawed milk must be used within 24 hours. Milk should never be refrozen.

+ Don't save any leftover heated milk longer then one hour; the saliva from the baby's mouth that may have gotten into the unused breast milk can cause bacteria to start growing.

How long should I breastfeed for each feeding?

How long a baby nurses depends on the baby. Some babies will be satisfied after ten minutes to a half hour on each side, and others simply like to take their time. The hour of the day or how long she had been asleep may make a difference. A baby who wakes up hungry after four hours of sleep may nurse longer and more vigorously than a baby who has slept for only two hours.

Some babies fall asleep at the breast and continue to use your breast as a pacifier. This habit can make your nipples very sore. It's a good idea to teach him that meal time is serious business. When your baby is hungry, nurse him until he seems to be losing interest, then burp him and offer the other breast. Nurse as before, but when he starts to play around or falls asleep, take him off the breast. If he's still fussy you can entertain him with other things; mealtime is officially over.

When you place your baby to breast let him suck on that breast until he stops or pulls away. It's good to have each side emptied before you burp, change the baby's diaper, and place him on the other breast.

Does it make any difference which breast I use first?

When you put your baby to breast, alternate which side you offer first. If you start with your left breast, for instance, baby will begin feeding with good long draws and most likely drain that breast completely of milk. When you switch to the right breast she'll be less hungry, her draw won't be as strong, and she probably won't drain it. So with the next feeding, start with the right breast to ensure that both breasts are emptied regularly. To keep track of which breast you last started with, pin a safety pin to that side of your bra. When the next feeding time comes along, start on the opposite breast. Don't forget to move the pin!

What about baby spitting up and hiccupping?

It's common for babies to spit up during and after feedings. Some babies spit up more readily than others. It's usually nothing to worry about unless your baby chronically vomits in a forceful manner—then it's time to call your pediatrician. If your baby does spit up too readily, here are a few things you can do to help:

+ Feed baby in a quiet, calm, and peaceful surrounding.

+ Avoid bright lights or interruptions.

+ Hold baby upright during a feeding.

+ Burp the baby at least twice during a feeding.

+ Keep baby in an upright position after the feeding.

+ Do not jostle or vigorously play with baby right after a feeding.

Hiccupping during feedings is also very common behavior, but you can continue feeding right through them. In fact, repeated swallowing will most likely cure them.

How can I be sure my baby is getting enough milk?

Count wet diapers. He should have at least six a day, with pale yellow urine. He should also have several small bowel movements throughout the day. Sleeping well between feedings and steady weight gain after the first week postpartum are also signs of a healthy intake.

For the first six months, breastfed babies don't need water, vitamins, or iron as long as they are breastfeeding well. Ask your pediatrician about fluoride and vitamin D supplements at his six-month checkup.

What should I know about my own intake of drugs and medications as well as my diet while breastfeeding?

Some medications aren't safe to take during breastfeeding. Be absolutely sure your doctor knows you are breastfeeding before he prescribes any medications. Also ask him about any over-the-counter medications you may be taking. For instance, Sudafed™ and any cold medications that dry up nasal congestion will also dry up your milk supply.

Some birth control pills might affect your milk production. Birth control pills inhibit the hormone that releases breast milk to the nipple.

Remember that caffeine is also a drug and can make the baby irritable and a poor sleeper. It can also build up in the baby's system, causing addiction. Alcohol and tobacco also can harm baby when you're breastfeeding. Nicotine is passed to the baby through breast milk, resulting in nicotine shock, vomiting, diarrhea, and rapid heart rate. Secondhand smoke is also dangerous. Never smoke around children, especially newborns. Studies show smoking increases the risk of sudden infant death syndrome (SIDS). 30–40% of all cases of SIDS could be prevented if the number of pregnant women who smoke could be reduced from 30% to zero. SIDS can be added to the list of other detrimental effects of maternal smoking during pregnancy, including increased risk of preterm birth, fetal mortality, childhood cancers, childhood allergies, infantile febrile seizures, birth defects of the urinary tract, and lower IQ. [1]

A short list of common drugs that have adverse effects on breastfeeding includes bromocriptine, cocaine, cyclophosphamide, cyclosporine, doxorubicin, ergotamine, lithium, methotrexate, phencyclidine (PCP), and Phenindione.

Although it should go without saying, illegal drugs have extremely dangerous effects on the nursing baby. Below are some of them and their effects on babies.

+ amphetamines: irritability, poor sleeping patterns

+ cocaine: intoxication and addiction

+ heroine: tremors, restlessness, vomiting, poor feeding habits

+ marijuana: only one report in literature; no effect mentioned

+ phencyclidine: possible hallucinations.

Whatever you eat, the baby eats too. If you eat gas-producing or spicy foods, your baby may become fussy and difficult to console. Sometimes it's difficult to tell if a baby is colicky or reacting to something you ate. If your baby becomes fussy for no apparent reason, try to remember what you ate for the past few meals. If it was something new, you may find it doesn't agree with the baby's digestive system. If you can't figure out exactly what may be causing the baby's problem, change to a fairly bland diet and then gradually increase new food items. Meanwhile, take comfort: babies who are reacting to a food in your diet usually resolve their discomfort in 24 hours.

Sometimes a baby will be allergic to dairy in your diet. This allergy could cause diarrhea, rash, fussiness, or gas within a few minutes or up to two hours after you ate a dairy food. If you suspect that dairy foods might be a problem, eliminate them from your diet for two weeks, then gradually reintroduce a dairy food while closely monitoring your baby's reactions.

Tell me about maternal illness and breastfeeding.

Your illness does not necessarily mean you'll have to wean your baby. In fact, if you have the flu, a cold, or a bacterial infection, just the opposite is true—be sure to continue to breastfeed because your baby will get the antibodies your body is producing. If you stopped breastfeeding, your baby could get sick too. If you're too ill to nurse, pump your milk and have your partner feed the baby with a bottle.

Some infectious diseases, such as HIV or untreated tuberculosis, preclude breastfeeding because they can be transmitted through breast milk to the baby. Mothers with hepatitis B can breastfeed only if their baby has had the hepatitis B vaccine within the first few days postpartum. There's no evidence of hepatitis C being transmitted to babies through breast milk. Of course, whatever the disease, always consult with your physician.

Mastitis is a bacterial infection of the breast caused by a blocked milk duct. Symptoms are swelling, burning, redness, and pain, and the mom usually feels feverish and sick. Physicians usually treat it by prescribing rest, warm compresses, breast support, antibiotics, and continued breastfeeding. Frequent nursing helps unclog the milk duct and drain the breast, preventing any spread of the infection. Baby will not be harmed.

I loved breastfeeding my babies. The convenience alone was a wonderful advantage, and the short- and long-term health benefits to both baby and mother are priceless. The way it permitted me to stop several times a day, settle into a comfortable couch with my feet up, and nuzzle my daughter to my breast to eat was wonderful, and it laid the foundation for a life-long bond between us.

Breastfeeding

Breastfeeding is an art that must be learned, and for some it may take a lot of work in the beginning. You may need assistance in getting started, emotional support after you've established breastfeeding, and people willing to lend a helping hand (figuratively speaking). This worksheet is designed to help you get information, learn what you want or need from others, and guide you through the months that you'll have your baby at breast.

First, like all the other worksheets, you'll need phone numbers of people who can help you. To start your list you'll need the numbers of your:

+ pediatrician _____
+ health clinic _____
+ birth center _____
+ hospital family birth center _____
+ midwife _____
+ family practitioner _____

Below are some phone numbers and/or websites of organizations that can help you find other professional help in your area:

La Leche League — 1-800-LALECHE (1-847-519-7730). Tell them what state and city you live in and they'll give you a number of a local leader.

International Board of Lactation Consultants — 1-703-560-7330. Or logon to their website at www.iblce.org.

International Lactation Consultant Association — www.ilca.org.

Write down any contacts that you found here:

Name _____

Phone Number _____

Address _____

Name _____

Phone Number _____

Address _____

Name _____

Phone Number _____

Address _____

Name _____

Phone Number _____

Address _____

Okay, now that you've collected the phone numbers and you're getting close to your due date, you'll need to make some decisions for your breastfeeding adventure.

This worksheet will let you put a lot of information on a couple of pages for an easy-to-access outline of what's important to you and how you'll want to proceed. It includes questions that lactation professionals usually ask, so have it handy before you make any calls.

Circle and/or check the answers, write comments all over the place, and at the end write out your own thoughts, concerns, and questions that I may have missed.

Coming Home With Baby

Before you come home with your baby you'll most likely have already had some instruction at the hospital (or from your midwife if you had a homebirth) that will help reinforce the points below. For now though, go through each of them so you'll be ready for any questions.

	Yes	No
1. I want to exclusively breastfeed my baby.	❏	❏

2. If I supplement, it will be _____ feedings per day.

3. My reason for supplementing is _____.

4. Because I'm breastfeeding, I know I don't need to give my baby a bottle. But if I decide to I'll start my baby on a bottle at _____ weeks of age. I'll do this _____ times a day.

   Remember: It's a good idea to breastfeed for at least 6 weeks before you offer a bottle so baby won't refuse the breast. Also, this could trigger the weaning process.

5. I plan to start my baby on solids at _____ weeks of age. My choices of solids are _____.

   Note: To help control the sweet tooth in later toddler-years, it's best to start with veggies.

6. I have a special place where I want to breastfeed   ❏   ❏
   my baby. It is _____.
   Hopefully someplace cozy, quiet, and very special.

7. My partner's job in breastfeeding my baby will be
   _____.

8. I am taking medication. It is _____.
   My physician/midwife knows this and it won't have any effect on my baby.

   Whenever you go to the doctor be sure he knows you're breastfeeding—it can change the way he prescribes medication.

WORKSHEET ❖ BREASTFEEDING

	Yes	No

9. I don't smoke. ❏ ❏

If you do smoke, please wash your hands and change your blouse before you snuggle your baby. This is also true if you have company or your partner smokes. Nicotine stays on your clothes and body and transfers to the baby.

10. I am not planning to offer my baby a pacifier. ❏ ❏

Research shows that using a pacifier can cause some nipple confusion with your baby and interfere with breastfeeding. Also, since they're harder than a nipple, babies have a tendency to bite and chew on a pacifier and then do the same on your breast. Talk about OUCH!

Breastfeeding and the Workplace

1. I'm going back to work in ＿＿ weeks/months.

2. My partner has ＿＿ weeks/days off until he returns to work.

   Laws are changing and many businesses are giving fathers up to 6 weeks off.

3. My workplace allows nursing breaks and will let someone bring my baby in every 4–5 hours. ❏ ❏

   If there isn't a private area at your workplace to nurse, then you'll have to make arrangements to meet your friend somewhere else.

4. I won't be able to breastfeed during working hours, so I'll need to pump my breasts. ❏ ❏

5. I don't have breast pump equipment or know how to use it. ❏ ❏

   Organizations in your area can help you find a breast pump to buy or rent and teach you how to use it properly.

	Yes	No

6. I have a private place at work where I can pump. ❏ ❏

Check the policy of your workplace on this. I'm sure that if they don't allow nursing, they have to at least provide a private location for you to pump.

7. I have a place to store my breast milk at my workplace. ❏ ❏

If you don't have a safe place to store your breast milk then you'll need to bring a cooler and some crushed ice to keep it fresh until you can get it home.

Nursing a Preemie

The most important thing to remember about nursing a preemie weighing less than six pounds is that—no matter what else happens—*she'll need your breast milk every 3–4 hours*. Here's a checklist to help you accomplish this.

1. I will pump at least 8–12 times a day. ❏ ❏

To be sure you can leave an adequate amount of milk in the nursery you will need to pump every 2–3 hours while you're awake.

2. I have discussed any medications that I am taking with my physician. ❏ ❏

Your premature baby's system is much less mature than a full-term baby's and won't be able to tolerate some medications.

3. Although I'm waking my baby every 3–4 hours to feed, if she wakes up earlier I'll offer my breast. ❏ ❏

4. If I come home before my baby I will get a fresh supply of breast milk to the nursery every day. ❏ ❏

Friends and family may be able to help you with this.

5. My baby has _____ wet diapers a day. I understand she should have a wet diaper for every feeding and at least one stool a day. ❏ ❏

Long Term Nursing

Here are the supplies you will need for breastfeeding.
Check off as you purchase them.

❑ a nursing bra with good support

❑ an electric breast pump with extra bottles, and/or a hand
breastfeeding pump, also with extra bottles

❑ plastic freezer-safe nursing bottle inserts for storing pumped milk

❑ nursing pads for inside your bra

❑ a "nursing pillow"
(it circles your middle and holds baby in position)

❑ breast shields for inverted nipples

❑ lanolin cream for nipples

❑ a portable cooler for storing pumped milk when you're away
from home

❑ a baby sling for nursing in public

That's about it for long term. When baby is hungry until about 7–8 months old, all you'll need to do is offer a breast. It's so convenient, free, easily digested, and a quick fix for those fussy times (especially when you're at the movies).

Use the space below to write any other issues you may want to discuss with your care provider regarding your breastfeeding experience.

_____

_____

_____

_____

_____

_____

11

Birthing Wisdom From Across The Country

◆

WWW... Wise Women on the Web

"Kind words can be short and easy to speak, but their echoes are truly endless."
—Mother Teresa

T his chapter of the book should be a lot of fun to read. It's filled with tidbits of information that I've received via email from doulas, midwives, childbirth educators, MDs, RNs, hypnotherapists, reflexologists, acupressurists, moms, and many others that answered my plea for tips and tricks on birthing. Through these emails I met lots of wonderful women completely dedicated to the art of birthing. I've included their names; you may recognize some of them (including yours truly). Some have websites; I hope you have as much fun looking over them as I did.

I want to thank everyone who took the time and patience to email me and share some of their techniques from their practice.

Please share these with the caregiver you have chosen and see if she is willing to try them too.

About Doulas

"I think something that should be mentioned is the possibility of how doulas create change in the way women are treated during their baby's birth and how our society views birth. This includes how doulas help in empowering women to feel like they had a choice or control in their birth. The increase in support leads to happier moms and happier babies, and thus happier families and a happier society. I think support and birth is where it can all start. A study by Penny Simkin talks about how mothers had better positive birth experiences if they felt like they had a choice and were supported. I can't remember all she said but it is awesome."

—*Blue Bradley*

"I have found that if the mother knows there is somebody with her that has the knowledge of what is happening and what to do about it, it helps her feel safe and calm."

— Sandra Taylor

"A good doula is like a good mom: she nurtures independence and growth, not dependence on her."

— Myra Lowrie

"A person fluent in Greek told me once that the word doula actually means 'walking with a woman,' which is very fitting for birth. A doula refers to a woman experienced in childbirth who provides continuous physical, emotional, and informational support to the mother and her partner. According to researchers and authors Kennel and Klaus (1933), the presence of a doula may have the following benefits:

1. 25% shorter labor
2. 60% reduction in epidural requests
3. 30% reduction in analgesia use
4. 50% reduction in the cesarean rate
5. 40% reduction in oxytocin use
6. 40% reduction in forceps births"

— Sabine Omvik

Prenatally

"First and foremost I try to get an idea of the woman's past, especially any trauma in her life and her own mother's birthing experience. I don't pry, I just let my pregnant moms know that pregnancy and birth is a tremendous opportunity for growth. It can shave five years off their therapy bill if they can utilize the moment. I also tell them that unresolved major issues are going to come up and that it's best if they come out during the pregnancy instead of making the labor dysfunctional leading to more trauma or, at best, the use of medication to numb all feelings. If I do see dysfunction in labor, I try to keep birth trauma to a minimum by dealing with the physical problem. The mom may not be ready to deal with issues then, but a powerful birth experience might give her the strength she needs down the road."

—Gloria Squitiro

"I like to educate people before their birth about why they would want to avoid a cesarean, the REAL reasons for a cesarean, and if one is needed, what to expect during the cesarean. Such as: what it will look like in the room, what they will be doing to you, sounds you might hear, etc."

—Sarah McKay

"I find the prenatal time spent with moms is valuable. Developing trusting relationship between doula and mom is of utmost importance. Understanding her fears and concerns, wishes, hopes and desires, and empowering her is fundamental. Helping her to be an active participant in her birth enables the mom to have a more positive experience. If a mom feels loved, cared for, and respected she can discover her strengths and have a sense of fulfillment and satisfaction when remembering her birth."

—Holly Wiersma

Breathing Techniques

"I like to let the mother find what is working for them, be it slow breathing, moaning, sighing, mantra, etc. I don't think that patterned breathing/panting works very well for most moms."

—Brenda Lane

"She has to find her own breathing technique. However, a doula can help her refocus during hard contractions or redirect her breathing again if she loses oversight."

—Sabine Omvik

"There are many breathing techniques out there. It would do an expectant mom and her coach good to learn as many ways to breathe as possible. During labor, you may find that you jump from one to the other, as your needs change based on the strength, duration, and challenge of each state of labor. There is slow, easy abdominal breathing, light chest breathing, chanting, variable accelerated breathing, panting, combination breathing, scrambled breathing, and urge-to-push breathing. All of them work well, but it is up to the mom and her coach to educate themselves about all the different kinds of breathing so they have the most resources to choose from during the course of labor. Many childbirth educators teach these forms of breathing. You can also find some information by reading the many good labor and delivery books out there. Many doulas are also very well trained in helping mom to breathe well for relaxation and progress."

—Gina Acosta

"During the most intense contractions, use eye-to-eye contact [either she and her husband, or you (make sure your breath is sweet)]. Have her look into your left eye and you stare into hers (it's easier to focus on just one eye). This brings the intensity out between you, and stops her from being so focused on the uterus. Once this connection is established, she will look for you, or him, in the room to do this."

—Jennifer Schepper

"I take my cues from yogic breathing. I think it is important to breathe fully and to be steady with each breath."

—Julie Reams

"During the last part of first stage, if she wants to verbalize, have her say in a low voice (high tightens things up) "open," or "open cervix," or "ommm…" These all help those last few centimeters. You can say this with her, or without her."

—Sue O'Connor

"Have the mom, before labor, practice breathing in through her nose and out through her mouth when she is practicing her breathing techniques. This will prevent her mouth from drying out."

—*Breck Hawk*

"What I've found in my three years working as a doula is that deep, slow-paced breathing is very effective all the way through active labor. Rarely have I seen a need for any kind of patterned breathing in active labor. Even as a woman reaches transition labor and the body really starts to naturally breathe faster and lighter, it is our job as a doula to support her breathing. I strongly believe that keeping your breathing as simple as possible through your whole labor really brings much relief to the mother."

—*Jennifer Schepper*

"Breathing in a couple of drops of peppermint oil on a wet washcloth calms the stomach and helps mom ease into a more relaxed state if feeling nauseous."

—*Myra Lowrie*

Relaxation

"I love using Penny Simkin's roving body check in between contractions to make sure mom is relaxed. It's also a nice thing to teach fathers to do during pregnancy and a way he can help her relax during early labor while they are still at home together. The way to do this is by gently touching different parts of mom's body to see if they are relaxed. The shoulders, chest, fingers, neck—anywhere that she usually tenses up."

—*Brenda Lane*

"I was given some good advice when I had my first child, dealing with the first stage of labor. This is good, especially with first-time moms, and I have given it as advice to all my doula clients. When you're going through those hours of anxiousness awaiting the oncoming unknown, it's best to get your mind off it and get it on something else—something to occupy you and be a good distraction. I recommend making bread. If you're not a baker, it is a good time to try to figure it out; if you are one, then try something really different. Or pick a new and crazy recipe to try if you really don't want to tackle bread—something that takes hours to make really works well, and if it's a three- to four-hour process it helps moms to forget —often long enough to really help them get on with labor."

—*Kari Shelton*

"When I was doing home births in Canada, I would have the moms make a birthday cake in the early stages of labor. Then after the birth we all settled in talked about the labor and birth and enjoyed the baby's first birthday cake."

—*Breck Hawk*

"Birth ball, birth ball, birth ball. My experience seems to include a lot of ability for moms to relax best on the ball, sitting in front of her doula or dad, having their neck and shoulders rubbed, and the other person (dad or doula) sitting in front of them. I also find that a lot of expectant moms do great with relaxation if they labor in the baby's room."

—*Jeannine Albertine*

"Relaxation is important during labor because it helps dilation—but that is easier said then done. Visualization sometimes helps, massage therapy, aromatherapy, distractions, encouragement, music, etc...."

—*Sabine Omvik*

"Get into some water! Massage, movement, focusing, and deep breathing."

—*Tara Beasley*

"The thing that works best for me and my clients is to teach them to totally sink into the bed, one muscle at a time. I help them make their body stay relaxed, each and every muscle, and I teach them to do the roaming body check with their partner. This is where the partner learns to watch for tension anywhere in her body. When the partner sees, for example, the shoulders tensing up, he then touches the shoulders and that is the woman's cue to totally drop her shoulders and make them relax."

—Julie Thompson

"One must make sure to remain relaxed, not only in the body but also in the mind, during labor. If one harbors tension or fear, they are telling their body that there is a dangerous environment for the baby to be born into and the muscle of the uterus will actually become rigid in order to stall the birth. If this happens, the uterus has to work against itself in order to dilate the cervix. It can cause labor to take longer, can create very real pain, and can also create complications, such as failure to progress as well as fetal distress, both of which could lead to unnecessary cesarean section. The solution: work hard before labor begins to counteract the negative effect of fear as it relates to labor and delivery. During labor, have support persons there to help you remain relaxed in all your muscles as well as relaxed and confident in your mind."

—Kelly Townsend

"When moms have trouble relaxing during labor, rhythmic movement is something that often helps… Or swaying from side to side while on one's knees, leaning over a birth ball or couch, often assists the mother to relax her buttocks, thighs, and pelvic floor—key areas to relax to facilitate labor."

—Karen Kohls

"When mom is having trouble dealing with her contractions, I tell the coach to consider a couple of things to help her become more relaxed and comfortable. How long has it been since she's urinated? If it's been more than an hour, you need to get her to use the bathroom. Most moms are hooked up to an IV with a lot of fluid running, so you have to consider she needs to void frequently. With all the pelvic pressure of labor, mom typically misses the cues of a full bladder and only notices that she's very uncomfortable all of a sudden.

"Also look at her environment to see what you can do to help her. Is it too warm or cold in the room? Is it too bright? Would she like a window opened for more light? Perhaps she'd like some soothing music.

"Think about all the senses—touch, smell, sight, sound, and taste. Address each one to see if there's something you can do to change the environment more to her liking. Check mom's position. How long has she been in that position? Perhaps you should suggest a change. This greatly helps with progress, and typically makes it more comfortable for mom. And consider her relaxation level. This is where massage and touch relaxation come into play. Might she need more pillows? Check her out emotionally. Consider what else you might need to try to help her become more relaxed and less tense."

—*Gina Acosta*

"I like to watch Penny Simkin's video on comfort measures at my clients' prenatal visit. I use the knee press, double hip squeeze, and forehead pressure at every birth. Something else I found effective is encouraging the mom to breathe with an open throat, or keep her throat open. I try to either breathe low with her or keep encouraging her until her breathing is releasing instead of tightening."

—*Gwen Peters*

Father's Role

"I have noticed that fathers sometimes want to rescue moms from the pain of labor, and that talking about that ahead of time can really help once labor is underway. Letting him know that his desire to 'save' her is a wonderful impulse that is awakened in labor so that he can be a better father once their baby is born, that that protectiveness is really the father in him being born. Mom actually doesn't need to be 'rescued' from her labor, just allowed to continue with as little interference as possible, and that he can best protect her by protecting her space, keeping the lights low, making sure no one chit-chats during a contraction, and keeping interruptions to a minimum."

—*Heather Baek*

"Father's role—very important! Encouragement, love for your partner, telling her how strong she is."

—*Sabine Omvik*

"I think that sometimes, because of our knowledge as birthing professionals and the ease we feel with it, we tend to be too much help. We need to remember that we are there to support and help the laboring mom, but we must also remember that we are not there to replace the father. Our job is to be available when it becomes too overwhelming to the father so he can just nurture his partner—this is where we are the strongest."

—*Breck Hawk*

"I have found that by having dad or partner help with massage, visualization, position changes, etc.—really having them take part in the birthing process—helps them not feel left out, and the mom feels a deep sense of comfort and support."

—*Maryanne Savino*

Mom's and Doula's Birth Bags

"I have some suggestions for mom's birth bag.

+ A water bottle with a stationary straw so moms between contractions don't have to strain to get a drink of water

+ A hair tie, because you will get hot

+ Lip balm for your lips is a must because of all the hard work and breathing

+ I carry a bottle of peppermint oil in my pocket in case a mom has nausea; it helps them a lot. I also carry peppermint candies so they can suck on something quickly and give them a boost of energy.

+ Warm socks, the kind with grips on them for walking and for keeping feet warm"

—*Ramona Majewski*

"I carry a small plastic wash basin in my bag, with peppermint salts for foot soaks, followed by rubs. This is especially relaxing before things get too tense."

—*Linda Cameron*

"I bring a camcorder and leave it on during private time so mom and dad can make beautiful pictures for the future. One of the most touching I have seen was in the hospital while the nurse was out of the room and I went for ice. The tenderness dad showed was forever captured on film."

—*Linda Cameron*

"I have a Rubbermaid stool that I leave in the van when I get to the house. If there is no stool available, I bring it in for dad to sit on when mom is in the bath, for mom to use when she is on her hands and knees, and for me to help my poor aching back."

—*Linda Cameron*

"I bring Astroglide® with me for women with vaginal dryness. It is essential to help slip that head out with some gentle swipes on the entire entrance to the vagina. It does what it says. Astroglide works wonders, and I haven't seen any tearing either."

—Kathleen Ruggio

"Having peppermint oil in my backpack allows me to put a couple of drops on a wet washcloth. I have the mom breath it in and this calms her stomach and helps mom ease into a more relaxed state if feeling nauseous."

—Ramona Majewski

Mother and Baby Massage

"Whether a mom is laboring naturally or with medication, I like to offer a foot massage while mom keeps her feet in a basin of warm water. Mothers find the water soothing and the foot massage relaxing, and she benefits from the necessity of being in a gravity-enhancing position when she sits up to receive the massage. Sometimes just pouring the water from a cup onto her feet is all she needs to relax. The gentle touch of water and the sound of it pouring can either follow or create a peaceful rhythm for the mom."

—Connie Sultana

"Massage therapy during labor: Counter-pressure on the glute muscles is a favorite of most of my moms. Also, a lot of shoulder rubs between contractions. One mom loved to breathe out a contraction while having her shoulders squeezed and eased."

—Jeannine Albertine

"Massage therapy during labor: Some women love to have their feet massaged either with or without oil. The back is always helpful, whether you actually massage, using counter-pressure or opening the pelvis a little further by putting the inside of your hands right on top of the pelvic bones and pressing inward."

—Sabine Omvik

"In infant massage I feel it is very helpful to set the mood ahead of time by keeping my room warm, having low-level lights, and giving my new parents a sample of my oils during their first session. I usually teach my class in four sessions, which allows the parents time to practice and feel more comfortable with their new skills, and give them time to ask me questions. I include many handouts on current parenting topics. I especially emphasize that we must 'ask the baby's permission' to massage her. Many parents are quite surprised to learn that babies give non-verbal cues to indicate whether or not they are ready for a massage. And, it sets an example to the parents that they must learn to respect their children's bodies and individuality. One trick that I have learned through the years is that the parent should flex the back of the hand forward and downward in order to massage the hands. If the palm of the hand is massaged in an upward position, the baby's fingers will automatically grasp and tighten (grasp reflex), and this position will be much more difficult for the parent to massage."

—Anne DeMaria

"Lavender flower massage oil (first check to see if the mother likes the smell) is soothing and when other nurses or doctors come into the room it's a reminder to them that they are in a sacred space."

—Juliana Walker

"For moms who like massage, the good old foot massage remains a favorite."

—Myra Lowrie

"Baby massage—but never without asking the baby for permission! Grape seed or very pure oils only. Lots of stretching and leg pedaling. Toes to nose, etc."

—Jeannine Albertine

"I do massage therapy during labor—mostly firm massage on hands and feet. I do find that late in labor some women, though, do not like to be touched and I respect that."

—Brenda Lane

"I feel that massage helps move fluid through tissue and would aid more in the reduction of swelling (as in a swollen ankle—you would apply ice to reduce swelling and use massage to move the edema out). I think the warm compresses are very effective for pain relief during crowning, and I highly recommend them, but if you are discussing swelling, it may not make sense to offer these instead of massage. The doula should always press the warm compresses to her face or wrist before applying to the mom, to make sure they do not burn her bottom."

—Ramona Majewski

"I teach infant massage to my many clients. They enjoy using massage time as a way to deepen their bond with their baby. Many say that it is a great way for them to increase their understanding of their baby's cues. Infant massage has many wonderful benefits for the baby and the parents. It helps the baby release stress, which means more rest for the baby and for everyone else."

—Shanti Sunshine

Positions in Labor and Pushing

"I find that squatting during pushing and changing positions during labor helps with moving the baby down. It's amazing how often moms have to be gently reminded to put their chin down to push, so it's nice, as a doula, to be able to stand near mom's head and gently encourage her chin down while dad's holding hands or legs, and/or taking photos."

—Jeannine Albertine

"One thing I have found very helpful to moms with hemorrhoids during pushing is to give firm counter-pressure to the afflicted area with a cool cloth moistened with witch hazel."

— Shellie Moore

"Most first-time moms don't know where to push or which area of the perineum to use. One good trick is to have mom in a semi-reclining position with her legs up and pulled back as far as she can (requires help from the doula or family), and the doula or dad between mom's legs holding one end of a long bath towel while mom holds the other end. As the contraction begins mom tries to pull the partner to her. The action of pulling the towel towards her causes her to bear down, using the exact muscles needed to help her baby out."

— Lori Wiseheart

"Some clients find the bathroom a comforting place to be during the first stage of labor. One mother I worked with liked sitting on the toilet. The small bathroom was a safe feeling space for her (dark, cool and cave-like). She was drinking a lot and found on one of her many visits that she was able to open her pelvis and relax sitting there. We supported her with pillows and she rested there. She might also try sitting on a birth ball at the sink with upper body supported and belly hanging forward. Finally, the shower is a wonderful place to go when labor gets intense. Sit down on a stool. Stay as long as you want."

— Juliana Walker

"The peanut birthing ball works great when mom wants to stay in bed but has a posterior baby. She gets on all fours, rocking back and forth on the peanut birthing ball. Great trick for getting those babies to move into position."

— Myra Lowrie

"I've seen some great laboring on an exercise ball, especially since you can take it into the shower. Also, some incredible births standing or on hands and knees, and a particularly amazing, very quick, compound presentation with no tears I'm convinced was successful because of a standing/lying across the bed birth position that the mom used during pushing."

— Tara Beasley

"I think the most important part is what happens before labor starts and during early labor in terms of getting baby positioned in the most effective way. I try to get all moms to do the polar bear position (aka knee-chest) in the days and weeks before labor starts. When labor begins, do this position again. If after this there is any suspicion that baby might still not be optimally positioned — given indication of OP or asynclitic baby, like early rupture of membranes, irregular contractions, gushing of amniotic fluid with position changes — then trying the polar bear again can never hurt. As well, things like using cold on the back, heat on the front, not only helps with pain control but will help the baby turn more optimally."

— Kathy Montgomery

"I have had a great deal of success with having clients push in a variety of positions. I especially like using the 'double hip squeeze' (pressing the hips from behind) with mom positioned facing the head of the bed (the head of the bed is all the way up). This has helped turn a few posterior babies."

— Julie Reams

"It seems like I am at quite a few posterior labors, and I find the biggest help to be changing positions often during labor. I encourage the use of the birth ball to help with rotation as well as laboring on hands and knees. If the baby is still posterior for the pushing stage I recommend moving from hands and knees to squatting to facing the head of the bed and continuing to change after about four to five contractions."

— Julie Reams

"In a labor that is going nowhere, I try to get the mom into a tub of water so that she can easily get into a jackknife position (lying on side, top knee up to chest, bottom leg out towards back). The water helps mom relax enough so that baby can get into an optimal birth position. I have also used the homeopathic remedy to bring about change."

—Gloria Squitiro

"Picture a tube of toothpaste. What needs to happen to get the toothpaste out easily? Take the cap off and squeeze. In what order would you do these to be most efficient? Take the cap off first, right? When pushing, focus more on releasing your pelvic floor, then pushing, and your baby will be born more easily! Once your pelvic floor releases to allow the baby to descend, your uterus does most of the work of pushing your baby out."

—Karen Kohl

"I use the three-contraction rule and we discuss this in the prenatal visit. That is, when we try anything new, like a new position, she tries it for three contractions. We do not count the contraction when she moves either. If, at the end, that is not working then we try something else."

—Becca Cartledge

"First and foremost, do what feels right to the mother at that time—what is her body telling her to do? Next, how about trying different positions to see what feels good? I like side-lying during the second stage for moms who are tired with a long labor. Also good when babies need to rotate from OT to OA, which are positions of the baby's head while it is descending through the birth canal during delivery.

—Brenda Lane

"Positions I like are gravity-driven, like standing, squatting, or sitting, and gravity-neutral, like side-lying or hands and knees position for labor and pushing."

—Sabine Omvik

Prenatal Exercises

"Good prenatal exercises are the usual squatting, pelvic rocking, etc. I find Kegels aren't as useful to some women as they are led to believe (yes, for afterward healing; no, for labor/delivery), but bulging exercises are great for pushing. Also, most important I find is diaphragmatic breathing. My best breather was an operatic singer. She literally sang arias between contractions and it helped to bring the baby down."

—Jeannine Albertine

"My focus is on stretching and range of motion. I explain that during labor you may be required to use your upper body to pull yourself up, thus the importance of shoulder range of motion. I encourage tailor-sitting to help widen the pelvis. I stress the importance of Kegels, especially immediately postpartum, and explain the importance of doing them now and forever."

—Barbara O'Brien

Determining False Labor from Real, and When to Transport

"Braxton Hicks usually makes your whole belly rock-hard. Though it can go on for awhile, it may subside by drinking something and lying down. Real contractions are usually felt lower in the belly, or even your back, and they keep coming back—there are breaks in between but they won't stop."

—Sabine Omvik

"To determine false labor from true labor, in false labor the contractions don't change when you change your activity. They stay the same in intensity, length of time between contractions, and how long the contraction lasts. With real labor the contractions become more intense, are closer together and last longer.

—Jeannine Albertine

"I encourage women to do the opposite of what they have been doing. If it is night and they have been sleeping, I encourage them to get up and shower. If it is day and they have been busy, try lying down, drinking fluids, and seeing what happens with the contractions."

—*Linda Sheppard*

"When a mom calls me with surges, I suggest drinking something hot and laying down; if they are false they'll usually stop."

—*Breck Hawk*

"If the contractions involve your WHOLE body (rather than just one part), it is labor!"

—*Brenda Lane*

"I always tell my clients to ask themselves this question: Why am I going to the hospital? Is it for medication? Because my partner says it is time to go? Because my contractions have been five minutes apart for the last two hours and are getting stronger? Because the shower at the hospital is better than ours? There are a number of answers and it's only [when you know them] that you can really evaluate the situation and decide on the correct course of action."

—*Rosemary Mason*

"When to transport? I always encourage my moms to stay at home until they no longer feel secure doing so. One mom didn't want to leave for the hospital, and dad wasn't feeling sure about it (contractions were four to five minutes apart, doc said go at five minutes, but the hospital was literally only four streets away and mom had BAD feelings about the doctor). Mom decided at three minutes apart to give in to dad's concerns and we transported. At the hospital, doc showed up, mom became highly emotional, blood pressure (which was normal in labor) went up—doc insisted on starting her on magnesium. The labor stalled for thirty minutes. The doc started talking cesarean, mom asked the doctor to leave. Trigger points and changed position helped restart labor, but it was very stressful experience for mom. Dad has now promised all future births that MOM decides when she feels it's time to transport."

—Jeannine Albertine

"Learning when it's time to transport mom is one of the most confusing issues for many moms and coaches. This is what I advise those in my childbirth classes: Educate yourself to know the emotional and physical sign points for each stage of labor. You should be comfortable with knowing what to expect in each stage as far as how mom is acting/reacting and what she feels. When mom is no longer able to walk, talk, and breathe through a contraction, needs continual support, and is becoming very serious, grumpy, and tired between contractions, it is probably a good time to go. The tendency with first-time moms in particular is to go to the hospital too early. Remember that you want to stay at home as long as you comfortably can to allow for the best relaxation and movement. Also consider that if you have orders for medication it's not in mom's best interest to use them until she's at 5 centimeters to avoid the possibility of her labor stalling and going off track. Monitor mom, watch how she's handling contractions, how she's feeling and acting emotionally, what's happening physically, how long the contractions are lasting, and how far apart they are. When it all comes together, it is time to go."

—Gina Acosta

Labor Management
at Home and Hospital

"Think of each contraction as important. Each one gets you closer to having the baby so you can welcome it. When a contraction reaches its peak, it hurts the most for only about 10 seconds and then it starts to come down. Contractions always end and then you get a break."

—Alice Gilgoff

"Know as much as you can about all of the different pain medications given during labor. Nurses don't have the time to explain all of them and they will give mom a choice as to which she wants to receive. If we as doulas know what each is and the effect on mom and baby, we can explain in detail these medications."

—Kim Killackey

"The first of two redeeming virtues I have as a doula are my calm and reassuring voice. My moms constantly tell me that as long as they can hear me they are fine. Part of this includes the roving body check. I will place my warm and calm hand on a visually tense area and then begin to use my voice to help her release and let go with her breath. My second virtue is my involvement of my coaches. When I am with a couple, I can quickly access what the coach is doing and guide him to provide comfort measures that help and not annoy the birthing woman."

—Ann Johnson

"For slower labor, sit at the end of the bed, put your thumbs in the middle of mom's feet, under the pads below the toes, and pull energy down through her body and out your hands, then down your spine and legs to the earth through your feet. Use your imagination to see this downward flow. If this is too New Age for your client, you don't have to tell her what you are doing. This downward flow of energy helps babies come down. Breathe with her through contractions as you do this."

—Sue O'Connor

"When mom wants to discuss a procedure or drug with me she asks the staff to leave while she 'discusses options with her husband.' The staff then feels more agreeable then if she says, 'discuss with my doula.' I remind my moms I am there to support them in having their birth experience."

—Myra Lowrie

"I have a great deal of success with Penny Simkin's 'Take Charge Routine.' When the mother is frustrated and feeling defeated I make sure that I ground her (usually by placing one hand on her shoulder). I make eye contact and hold it, and then I tell her to breathe with me while I lead her with breathing and encouraging words through the contraction. It is amazing to see how calming and grounding it is for a distraught woman."

—Julie Reams

"I teach parents while I doula them. I have a pocket-size pelvis model, with a baby with the cord and placenta, etc., so I show them when they have back labor and the need to change positions. I also have an anatomy coloring book with pages that I ask them to color while we learn about baby and birth. It works well with teens and women that had only elementary or some years in high school."

—Sr. Gladys Leigh

"Warm packs to the perineum when completely dilated and starting to push really helps, even with an epidural; they can still feel the warmth and relax."

—Sr. Gladys Leigh

"Even a shower in a hospital with no tub is helpful."

—Becca Cartledge

"To turn a posterior baby, place ice packs on the mother's back and the baby turns away from them. I have seen this work a couple of times."

—Dena Carmosino

"Moms sometimes get it in their head that the way they have seen it in the movies and on TV is the way to have a baby — either lots of drugs, or if they relax enough, they can get the baby out. This sometimes works, but for a number of women, moaning, groaning, and screaming is what gets their baby out. That is okay too. I would encourage moms to think about how they deal with pain on a daily basis; does she take a deep breath and relax when she stubs her toe, or does she hop up and down and say ouch? A wonderfully holistic way to prepare for a birth is with the book series called *Birthing From Within*, which can be reached at www.birthingfromwithin.com."

—*Augustine Daniels*

"At-home pain management: massage, breathing, ice. Rice socks with rice, lavender, chamomile, cinnamon, and peppermint heated in the microwave are a huge hit with my moms. In fact, sometimes my dads like to use them for a sore back if mom is resting. Also, the bathtub is a definite favorite.

"In-hospital pain management: Same as at home, however some moms do at that point decide on meds. If they do, a low-dose epidural seems to be about the best choice for most moms. Narcotics can allow them to doze, but will have them wake up unable to 'get on top' of their contractions."

—*Jeannine Albertine*

Induction

"Natural induction: Evening primrose oil applied directly to the cervix; sex; and nipple stimulation. One option that I've had good success with is the use of massage, targeting the uterine contraction points (around the heel of the foot, the baby toe, above the ankle, top of the shoulders, and top of the head). I use massage oil that is a blend of pure essential oils from jasmine, cinnamon leaf, and peppermint in a pure carrier oil base."

—*Jeannine Albertine*

"I have thoroughly researched castor oil and evening primrose oil as tools to aid in labor induction and cervical ripening respectively."

—*Bonu deCaires*

In the Hospital

"What happens in the hospital: I find that unprepared parents tend to be scared by the equipment, and dads sometimes become fascinated by the monitors and focus more on the machine than on their partners.

"Monitoring in hospital: In one experience at Cedar's, mom was told she must be monitored (externally) for 20 minutes out of each hour. The staff was so wonderful, however, they allowed her to be monitored while sitting on the birth ball in front of the monitor for 20 minutes. The freedom from the monitor gave her time for walks and showers."

—*Jeannine Albertine*

Birth Plans

"One of my many doula tricks includes the birth plan. I have found through the years that some care providers like them and some do not. There are now many websites offering birth plans that you can formulate online. My advice is to check out these sites and, with your doula, present a checklist of issues and concerns for the way you want your labor to be. We start out with a nice 'fluffy' polite thank-you paragraph, then a list of wishes. All of the above desires are with the knowledge and understanding (which is stated) that birth can change in a moment's notice so the bottom line would be the health and wellbeing of the mother and baby. I have stopped calling them birth plans, because of the almost-expected comment of, 'This is a C-section waiting to happen'; I now call them 'desire lists' or 'wish lists,' which also helps the mother to not to be set up emotionally if things do not go as planned. When taking this plan into the care provider to review, it is helpful for the doula to be there too. The care provider should be asked to sign or initial the plan, which then goes into the client's chart."

—*Cindy Morris*

"One thing I tell all my clients is that they are in charge of their birth and their bodies. As a doula, I will make sure all their wishes are fulfilled as stated in their birth plan."

—*Fran Slafky*

"If you want all your birth attendants to remember what you want for your birth, then write it down. It's way too much information for anyone to remember after talking to you weeks before, and way too much information to tell people while in the midst of labor. A birth plan is a communication tool for all of the people who might care for you during labor. In a hospital, most, if not all those people, will not have met you before."

—*Karen Kohl*

"Ask the doctor or midwife to not give any injections of numbing agents into the perineum during the pushing phase, as often occurs. The fluid they inject definitely causes edema and therefore gives the tissue less flexibility."

—Shellie Moore

"Make sure you have gone over your birth plan with the doctor that is going to deliver your baby. Communicate any concerns, fears, and anything you feel strongly about. Ask the doctor to initial your birth plan so you will not run into problems in the hospital."

—Rosie Ruiz

"If your desire is to have a natural birth, find a care provider that is more than lip service. Many will say, 'Oh yes, I will be happy to follow your birth plan,' and walk out in the hall and laugh at the idea of having a natural birth. Clarify what you mean by natural birth—vaginal, without drugs, manipulation, augmentation, or intervention. Find a care provider who is EXPERIENCED in natural birth. Ask, 'How many babies have you delivered naturally?' 'Over intact perineum?' 'What positions have you delivered babies in other than with mom on their back with feet in stirrups?' 'What is your C-section rate?' 'Epidural rate?' Your chances of having the birth choices honored increase drastically when you choose a care provider who is respectful, experienced, and SUCCESSFUL in natural birth."

—Linda Weaver

"In the discussion of birth plans I really encourage [the parents] to discuss this with every doctor in the group. Of course, I ask for a copy of the birth plan because sometimes that is the only one that seems to make it to the hospital."

—Becca Cartledge

"Please remind moms to be flexible. There's an old joke: If you want to make God laugh, tell him your plans. They are great as a guideline, and always get them signed by the doctor. That way anything that differs from hospital policy is already okayed by the doctor, however flexibility is definitely the key in my experience."

—Jeannine Albertine

Breastfeeding

"For a first encounter with breastfeeding (positions, aids for sleepy babies and moms) lots and lots of pillows are great help. The football hold seems to be best for post-C-section moms. The best advice I can share: Make sure baby's mouth is WIDE open before attempting to latch on. That way a large area is in the mouth and there is less likelihood of sore nipples. Also, air dry after feeding—and if nipples get sore after milk has come in use a drop or two of the milk to soothe the nipples."

—Jeannine Albertine

Herbs in Pregnancy and Labor

"I encourage ladies to use herbs in their labors pre-natally and with breastfeeding. Red raspberry is an herb that can be used pre-natally for good uterine function and tone. Blue or black cohosh can be used to augment or induce labor. Blessed thistle can be used to stimulate lactation while nursing."

—Donna Leach

"I have a great article on the HUGE benefits of alfalfa, also spirulina is great if it works well for your constitution and doesn't cause constipation."

—Tara Beasley

"I have found when a mom is 'stuck' at a certain dilation there is a homeopathic arnica that can help when applied to the cervix. I have seen two women stuck at 5 cm for hours; as soon as we applied the arnica they were able to complete dilation within 30 minutes. Rose oil applied counterclockwise to the belly is really good for turning breech babies or posterior babies. Peppermint oil is good for labor for headaches or nausea. Just having the mom smell it helps a lot. For morning sickness, take one to two drops and apply it to the back of the tongue. If a mother is having trouble urinating, put a few drops of peppermint oil in the toilet before she sits down."

— *Tara Tulley*

Acupressure

"In my experience, I have found that acupressure of bladder 67 (outside portion of the baby toe) is very useful in turning breech babies at around 34–36 weeks gestation. What I like about this method is that it is so non-intrusive, and the baby does not turn if the baby is unable to turn. I also find that this point is wonderful to stimulate during labor if the baby seems to doze off for too long and the labor is dragging because of it. One tip that may seem strange—but has been helpful—is that a mom with a breech baby can tape a grain of uncooked rice on that pressure point to assist in turning her own baby. I also use pressure point on the hand; the fleshy point between the thumb and the body of the hand is a great elimination point during labor."

— *Jeannine Albertine*

"I have great success in using acupressure to stimulate contractions and to help relieve labor pains. The spleen 6 point is very powerful and can induce contractions so it should not be used until the due date. The point is located about four finger-breadths above the inner ankle. The point should be pressed hard, with the thumb coming from behind the leg. It is generally a tender area and may hurt when pressure is applied correctly. Apply for about 15 seconds three times in a row with a few seconds of rest in between."

— Shanti Sunshine

"The two points I use most often are the L14—also known as the headaches point—and K3 (between the anklebone and Achilles tendon). I find that they are good for reducing panic and relaxing the mom."

— Brenda Lane

"There are two great acupressure points: Large Intestine 4, located on the back of your hand in the web between the base of your thumb and index finger, and Spleen 6, located four finger-breadths above your inner anklebone. Only use during labor and for a few on-off cycles lasting from 10 to 60 seconds."

— Sabine Omvik

HypnoBirthing® and Hypnosis

"In spite of HypnoBirthing, I have not found that hypnosis works as anesthesia during labor and delivery. In any case, my personal preference is to help mothers be more present and not to dissociate. I have found, however, that hypnosis works very well to help alleviate fears and mental obstacles, like the belief that a woman's mother and sister having a cesarean means that she is doomed to have one as well. Hypnosis also helps a woman to expend the minimum of energy during labor, not wasting as much on resistance, or muscle tension in secondary parts of her body. Hypnosis is also excellent for helping a mother bond with her baby even before birth, so that she is more connected and motivated throughout labor and in early postpartum to get to know her baby and feel like there is a team effort between them. I have also used hypnosis during delivery to increase the strength and frequency of contractions, to help a baby turn into a better position, or even to help calm a mother during a cesarean delivery."

—Chantal De Soto

"Although I have not had any formal training in hypnosis, I have specialized in storytelling to children and adults, and have enjoyed the success of that hobby for many years. Since being involved in labor support as a doula I have found guiding women and hubbies with creative visualization before, during, and after their birthing experiences as helpful as any other comfort measure."

—Deb MacFarlane

Music

"I use lots of music. I encourage clients to pick what works for them. In my personal first birth I used Bob Marley, but I don't expect many parents would be into that. My favorite CDs have been nature sounds, but also I love lullabies and classical music. I just got a CD that is called 'Chatter with Angels' under the label of Twin Sisters; it's African American lullaby music. It's wonderful—we all must be aware of cultural diversities. I also have Sarah McLaughlin, Mazzy Star, and Enya. With pushing, the music needs to be at a faster pace then the labor music.

"I encourage clients to explore music and find types of music that makes them feel good. I believe that, with music, clients have an easier time relaxing and they tend to move more; it actually seems to relax the staff also."

—Angel Turlington

"The most significant factor I have found very helpful as a doula is music. There are many calming CDs and tapes available, and most hospitals have players, but I bring my own just in case one is not available or is broken. You can use visual imagery of being at the beach and you can have the sound effects to go along too. Women really try and get into it because you're not just asking them to imagine but they feel as if they are there."

—Georgeanne Saddington

"I have found that sound and music are powerful allies to the doula work. Much of the work I do is closely related to music therapy and therefore not easily shared. But there are other practices such as 'toning' that can be practiced by everyone. The pregnant mothers I work with have found that making sounds and toning from deep within one's belly relaxes the cervix and the throat, allowing the expression of pain and joy to be expressed freely. Soothing music adds great comfort, and, in addition, the right music also assists with breathing and focuses the mind."

—Giselle Whitwell

Imagery

"Visualize what each contraction is doing, moving the baby down and out. Visualize the cervix like a flowering opening. Each contraction makes it open just a little bit more."

—Alice Gilgoff

"I find that imagery works much better when the mother practices it beforehand. I have the mothers go through their photo album and pick out pictures of their favorite things (sculptures, pets), relaxing moments, or ultrasound photo. I have them bring their favorite stuffed animal from the baby room or any object that energizes, relaxes, or motivates. I use these different objects or pictures when the labor has reached the point that they need that feeling. For example, when mom is pushing and feels that she can't go on, I use the ultrasound picture to remind her why she is doing this. If mom is getting tired of pushing, I will use a bright colored object or picture that is full of energy. If mom is cold, I will use a picture of the sun or a warm beach. Or if she is hot, I use pictures of a cool rain.

"Here is a quick little trick: When explaining what the cervix does during labor, use a lifesaver as the example. It starts off thick with just a little hole in the center, but as you have it in your mouth the thickness slowly starts to thin and the hole gradually opens up wider."

—Angela Rabenberg

Postpartum Doula

"Postpartum work for me is whatever you need—massage, creative visualization, hair styling, house cleaning, grocery shopping, rocking the baby, getting up in the middle of the night and bringing the baby to mom, changing diapers, taking care of the siblings, offering light help in breastfeeding, and cooking."

—Deb MacFarlane

"I bring each of our clients a gift bag, filled with samples, area parenting magazines, etc. I also include coupons for free copies of national magazines, like *Mothering*. The most appreciated thing in the bag is a batch of homemade cookies or bread. I bring a fresh-baked goodie each day I work with a client."

—Teri Bavley

"Postpartum things to have on hand that will save you.

1. Peroxide (removes blood in an instant, for panties, etc.)
2. Tucks
3. Witch-hazel (for the tucks)
4. Always maxi pads with wings 'overnight'
5. Carrot juice (to help the bowels move)
6. Big supply of raisins (same as above)
7. Oatmeal cookies and oatmeal (for the milk supply)
8. Breast pump (rental—hospital grade)
9. Throw away all formula so mom is not tempted in a moment of weakness when some well-meaning visitor asks if you're sure the baby is getting enough.
10. Hot packs (for the engorged breasts)
11. Washable breast pads, 100% flannel cotton
12. A sign on the front door: Do not disturb.
13. *So That's What They're For*, the best breastfeeding book available

"Call everyone and ask which night they will bring food after baby is born from 1–14 days. The day the baby is born, call #1 and she will call the following number. So when signing up each person, be sure they receive the phone number of the next person in line. When the baby is born this will be a nice way to relay the news and get the volunteers ready to prepare their dinners. Find a place in your area who does fluff and fold, and have the laundry sent out the first week. Ask a teenage girl if she wants to earn a little bit of money by doing some light housework for you. Ask each visitor to switch a load of laundry from the washer to the dryer and toss a new one in for you. Have the teenager fold and put away."

—*Kris Luitwieler*

"My primary focus is to help the mother (and partner) REST. I tell them that the one constant I have seen is sleep deprivation. I encourage the mom to sleep when I am there. I take care of the baby. I usually work with first-time moms, so they are not used to attachment parenting. I tell them that when they sleep with the baby and the baby moves, they'll wake up; when the baby doesn't move, they'll wake up. So they really sleep better initially when I am there. When I am gone, I encourage them to sleep together. I encourage and help with breastfeeding. I have great faith in women's bodies. I do minimum housework, but if the dishes in the sink or the baby's undone laundry is bothering mom, I'll take care of it. I want her to REST."

—*Ellen Richter*

"A suggestion for postpartum moms is to have a list of things to do on the fridge. When people come to visit keep it to a short visit (about five minutes), if they ask what they can do, show them the list and ask if they would like to pick something from the list and do it for you while they visit."

—*Heather Shelley*

Miscellaneous Tidbits

"Applying compresses, soaked in ice water and wrung out, to the perineum will work great to reduce swelling."

—*Brenda Lane*

"It helps to have a BIG bag of tricks, since I never know in advance what will work for each client in labor. Some of the tools I use are these:

- ✦ Positive encouragement (gives mom confidence in her body's ability to birth—fear and doubt can hinder labor progress)

- ✦ Water (can speed up labor and helps mom to relax)

- ✦ Atmosphere (dim lights, soft music, soft voices— whatever is a relaxing environment for you)

- ✦ Massage (most all moms LOVE this part)

- ✦ Aromatherapy (fragrances that help you relax, or give you energy, depending on what is needed at the moment)

- ✦ Birth ball (helps baby descend into the pelvis and align with pelvic outlet, also helps support perineum and is a comfortable place for mom to labor upright)

- ✦ Prayer (I believe that where we are limited, He is strong and is capable of doing what we cannot—BUT I want to be sensitive to YOUR desires and only use prayer if you tell me you are comfortable with it)

- ✦ Natural measures for inducing or augmenting labor (ONLY if induction is medically indicated by your doctor or midwife)

- ✦ Position changes (encourages endorphins, which give natural pain relief, encourages descent of baby, helps labor progress more quickly, aligns baby with pelvic outlet, etc.)

✦ Help with relaxation and visualization

✦ Hot/cold packs (ease discomfort and encourage relaxation)"

—Donna Leach

"I am using the *rebozo* (Mexican shawl) as a comfort measure for childbirth. The *rebozo* is a wonderful tool to be used to comfort labor women besides the well-known and traditional way to carry the baby. My website to view this is www.portaldemama.com."

—Guadalupe Trueba

"I give a copy of the pregnant patient's bill of rights, but I go over informed consent and what it really means. The questions are these:

When a test is suggested

✦ What is the reason for it?
  What problems are we looking for?

✦ What will it tell us?
  How accurate or reliable are the results?

✦ If the test detects a problem what happens next?

✦ If the test does not detect a problem, what happens next?

When a treatment or intervention is suggested

✦ What is the problem? Why is it a problem?
  How serious is it? How urgent is it that we begin
  treatment? What if we wait? What if we do nothing?

✦ Describe the treatment. How is it done?
  What are the alternatives? How are they done?

✦ If it does not succeed, what is the next step?

✦ What are the risks of the treatment?

"This list of questions is what they bring to the doctor appointments, and anytime they go to the hospital."

—Glenda Hamilton

"To relieve episiotomy pain and swelling, dampen a maxi-pad with water and place it in the freezer for a few hours. It will provide an ice pack that fits beautifully in your underwear and won't leak.

"One thing that I've used on more then one occasion is a Tupperware rolling pin. It sounds crazy, but the end comes off and I fill it with hot water and roll it on my mom's back. It works great for back labor. I have them stand and lean on the bed or their partner and I literally roll their back."

—Donna Marcosson

"Another thing that I always tell people to do is to bring cookies or something else for the nursing staff. The nurses are much more willing to give you what you want."

—Tara Tulley

"For a fearful momma, put your hand on her heart and visualize green for a few seconds."

—Sue O'Connor

12

Coalition for Improving Maternity Services

✦

And What an Improvement!

"There are two ways to live your life. One is as though nothing is a miracle. The other is as though everything is a miracle."
    —Albert Einstein

I'm dedicating this chapter to a powerful organization that's not only supported by a wonderful group of childbirth advocates, but is helping birth sites become much more birth friendly in the way they treat their clients.

The Coalition for Improving Maternity Services (CIMS—pronounced "kims") is made up of numerous individuals and more than 50 organizations representing over 90,000 members. The founding members included midwives, physicians, nurses, childbirth educators, labor support providers, lactation consultants, postpartum care providers, and consumer advocates. You can find the list of the organizations by visiting their website, MotherFriendly.org, and clicking on "The ratifying organizations of the Mother-Friendly Childbirth Initiative[1] are:"

Together, the founding members created the Mother-Friendly Childbirth Initiative, an evidence-based document that provides guidelines for identifying and designating mother-friendly birth sites, including hospitals, birth centers, and homebirth services.

CIMS' mission is to promote a wellness model of maternity care that will improve birth outcomes and substantially reduce the costs of birth—direct and indirect, short-term and long-term. This evidence-based mother-, baby-, and family-friendly model focuses on prevention and wellness as the alternatives to high-cost screening, diagnosis, and treatment programs.

The CIMS Principles

Normalcy of the Birthing Process

+ Birth is a normal, natural, and healthy process.

+ Women and babies have the inherent wisdom necessary for birth.

+ Babies are aware, sensitive human beings at the time of birth and should be acknowledged and treated as such.

+ Breastfeeding provides the optimum nourishment for newborns and infants.

+ Birth can safely take place in hospitals, birth centers, and homes.

+ The midwifery model of care, which supports and protects the normal birth process, is the most appropriate for the majority of women during pregnancy and birth.

Empowerment

+ A woman's confidence and ability to give birth and to care for her baby are enhanced or diminished by every person who gives her care and by the environment in which she gives birth.

+ A mother and baby are distinct yet interdependent during pregnancy, birth, and infancy. Their interconnectedness is vital and must be respected.

+ Pregnancy, birth, and the postpartum period are milestone events in the continuum of life. These experiences profoundly affect women, babies, fathers, and families, and have important and long-lasting effects on society.

Autonomy

Every woman should have the opportunity to:

✦ have a healthy and joyous birth experience for herself and her family, regardless of her age or circumstances;

✦ give birth as she wishes in an environment in which she feels nurtured and secure, and where her emotional wellbeing, privacy, and personal preferences are respected;

✦ have access to the full range of options for pregnancy, birth, and nurturing her baby as well as accurate information about all available birthing sites, caregivers, and practices;

✦ receive accurate and up-to-date information about the benefits and risks of all procedures, drugs, and tests suggested for use during pregnancy, birth, and the postpartum period, with the rights to informed consent and informed refusal; and

✦ receive support for making informed choices about what is best for her and her baby based on her individual values and beliefs.

Do No Harm

✦ Interventions should not be applied routinely during pregnancy, birth, or the postpartum period. Many standard medical tests, procedures, technologies, and drugs carry risks to both mother and baby and should be avoided in the absence of specific scientific indications for their use.

✦ If complications arise during pregnancy, birth, or the postpartum period, medical treatments should be evidence-based.

Responsibility

+ Each caregiver is responsible for the quality of care she or he provides.

+ Maternity-care practice should be based not on the needs of the caregiver or provider, but solely on the needs of the mother and child.

+ Each hospital and birth center is responsible for the periodic review and evaluation, according to current scientific evidence, of the effectiveness, risks, and rates of use of its medical procedures for mothers and babies.

+ Society, through both its government and the public health establishment, is responsible for ensuring access to maternity services for all women and for monitoring the quality of those services.

+ Individuals are ultimately responsible for making informed choices about the healthcare they and their babies receive.

Mother-Friendly and Baby-Friendly

The Initiative outlines ten steps for mother-friendly care and includes as a requirement that mother-friendly birthing services also qualify as baby-friendly according to the World Health Organization's guidelines.[2]

1. Have a written breastfeeding policy that is routinely communicated to all healthcare staff.

2. Train all healthcare staff in skills necessary to implement this policy.

3. Inform all pregnant women about the benefits and management of breastfeeding.

4. Help mothers initiate breastfeeding within a half hour of birth.

5. Show mothers how to breastfeed and how to maintain lactation even if they should be separated from their infants.

6. Give newborn infants no food or drink other than breast milk unless medically indicated.

7. Practice rooming in: allow mothers and infants to remain together twenty-four hours a day.

8. Encourage breastfeeding on demand.

9. Give no artificial teat or pacifiers (also called dummies or soothers) to breastfeeding infants.

10. Foster the establishment of breastfeeding support groups and refer mothers to them on discharge from hospitals or clinics.

Familiarizing yourself with these ten steps will help you decide if the facility you are considering as a birth site is one that is mother-friendly according to the CIMS guidelines.

First you must learn as much as you can about choices that will be available—or not available—to you while you are in labor and while you deliver your baby. Your birth professional/doula can help you with this because she has a lot of experience and knows what birth centers are offering in your area. Pick her brain before asking questions at the birth center.

Birthing care facilities that have proven themselves better and healthier for mothers and babies are called *mother friendly.* Some birth clinics or hospitals are more respectful and caring than others, and they offer more choices and are less likely to interfere and use interventions.

When you are deciding where to have your baby, you'll probably be choosing from different facilities, such as birth centers, hospitals, or homebirth centers.

A mother-friendly birthplace, according to CIMS, offers these ten steps from the mother-friendly initiative.

Mother-friendly hospital and birthing clinics will:

1. offer all birthing mothers

    + unrestricted access to the birth companions of her choice, including fathers, partners, children, family members, and friend;

    + unrestricted access to continuous and physical support from a skilled woman such as a doula or labor-support professional; and

    + access to professional midwifery care[3];

2. provide accurate descriptive and statistical information to the public about its practices and procedures for birth care, including measures of interventions and outcomes[4];

3. provide culturally competent care—that is, care that is sensitive and responsive to the specific beliefs, values, and customs of the mother's ethnicity and religion[5];

4. provide the birthing woman with the freedom to walk, move about, and assume the positions of her choice during labor and birth, and discourage the use of the lithotomy position[6];

5. provide clearly defined policies and procedures for

    + collaboration and consulting throughout the prenatal period with other maternity services, including communicating with the original caregiver when transfer from one birth site to another is necessary; and

    + linking the mother and baby to appropriate community resources, including prenatal post-discharge follow-up and breastfeeding support[7];

6. not routinely use practices and procedures that are unsupported by scientific evidence, including but not limited to the following:

   ✦ shaving,

   ✦ enemas,

   ✦ IVs,

   ✦ withholding nourishment,

   ✦ early rupture of membranes, or

   ✦ electronic fetal monitoring.

   Other interventions are limited as follows:

   ✦ has an induction rate of 10% or less;

   ✦ has an episiotomy rate of 20% or less with a goal of 5% or less;

   ✦ has a total cesarean rate of 10% or less in a community hospital and 15% or less in tertiary care hospitals; and

   ✦ has a VBAC rate of 60% or more with a goal of 75% or more[8];

7. educate staff in non-drug methods of pain relief and not promote the use of analgesic or anesthetic drugs not specifically required to correct a complication[9];

8. encourage all mothers and families, including those with sick or premature newborns or infants with congenital problems, to touch, hold, breastfeed, and care for their babies to the extent compatible with their conditions[10];

9. discourage nonreligious circumcision of the newborn[11]; and

10. strive to achieve the WHO-UNICEF "Ten Steps of the Baby-Friendly Hospital Initiative" to promote successful breastfeeding (pages 302, 303).

You should freely ask for and expect these provisions for your birth experience. Be aware of how open and willing the facility you are considering responds to your requests and concerns. You may want to ask some of the questions listed below to help you learn more.

Questions for You to Ask

Who can be with me during labor and birth?

Mother-friendly birth facilities accept that the birthing mother decides whom she wants to have with her during her birth. These people may include fathers, partners, children, other family members, and friends. They also accept that a birthing mother will be accompanied by a doula or labor-support person who is trained to help women cope with labor and birth. She never leaves the birthing mother alone. She encourages her, comforts her, and helps her understand what is happening in terms of labor and birth.[1]

What happens during a normal labor and birth in your setting?

Personnel at a facility that gives mother-friendly care will tell you how they handle every part of the birthing process. For example, find out how often they give a mother a drug to speed up the birth or if their policy is to allow labor and birth to happen on its own timing.[2]

They will also tell you how often they use certain procedures. For example, their records will reveal the percentage of cesarean sections they do every year. If the number is too high, you will want to consider having your baby in another place or with another doctor or midwife. Refer to the previously mentioned guidelines about rates of interventions. The rule of thumb is to carefully evaluate their induction, episiotomy, cesarean, and VBAC rates.

How do you allow for differences in culture and beliefs?

Mother-friendly birthplaces are sensitive to the mother's culture. They know that mothers and families have different beliefs, values, and customs.[3]

Can I walk and move around during labor? What position do you suggest for birth?

In mother-friendly settings, you can walk around and otherwise move about as you wish during labor. You can choose the positions that are most comfortable and work best for you during labor and birth. Mother-friendly settings almost never put a woman flat on her back with her legs up in stirrups for the birth.[4]

How do you ensure that everything goes smoothly when my nurse, doctor, midwife, or outside family-centered agencies must work with each other?

Ask, "Can my doctor or midwife come with me if I have to be moved to another place during labor?" and "Can you help me find people or agencies in my community who can help me before and after the baby is born?"

Mother-friendly places and people will have a specific plan for keeping in touch with the other individuals who are caring for you. They will talk to others who give you birth care. They will help you find people or agencies in your community to help you, from shelters, support groups, and breastfeeding support, to on-going health care if needed.[5]

What things do you normally do to a woman in labor?

Experts say some methods of care during labor and birth are better and healthier for mothers and babies, and medical research shows us which of them are the most beneficial. Mother-friendly settings only use methods that have been proven to be best by scientific evidence.[6]

Sometimes birthplaces use methods that are not proven to be best for the mother or her baby. For example, research has shown that it's usually not helpful to break the bag of waters to induce or speed up labor.

Following is a list of concerns you should ask about. These common procedures are not helpful and may even hurt healthy mothers and babies. They are not proven to be best for the mother or baby, and they are not mother-friendly.

✦ Continuous fetal heart rate monitoring: The baby's heart rate should not be monitored continuously with a machine. Instead, it is best to have your nurse or midwife listen to the baby's heart from time to time using a stethoscope.

✦ Breaking the waters: Your bag of waters should not be broken early in labor.

✦ Intravenous feeding: Nourishment by IV is rarely necessary.

✦ Forbidding eating and drinking during labor: You should be allowed to nourish and hydrate yourself to suit your body's needs.

✦ Shaving: This traditional practice is unnecessary.

✦ Enema: This traditional practice is also unnecessary.

A birthplace that uses these outdated and inappropriate procedures on the majority of mothers is not mother-friendly.

How do you help mothers stay as comfortable as they can? Besides drugs, how do you help mothers relieve the pain of labor?

The people who care for you should know how to help you cope with labor without resorting to drugs. They should suggest such things as changing your position, relaxing in a warm bath, having a massage, and listening to music. These strategies are called *comfort measures*.

Comfort measures help you handle your labor easily and help you feel more in control. The people who truly support you will not try to persuade you to use a drug for pain unless you need it to take care of a specific medical problem. All drugs affect the baby.[7]

What if my baby is born early or has special problems?

Mother-friendly places and people will encourage mothers and families to touch, hold, breastfeed, and care for their babies as much as they can. They will encourage this even if the baby is born early or has a medical problem at birth.

Do you circumcise?

Medical research disproves the need to circumcise baby boys. It is painful and risky. Mother-friendly birthplaces discourage circumcision unless it is for religious reasons.[9]

How do you help mothers who want to breastfeed?

The World Health Organization composed the following list of mother-friendly ways birthplaces support breastfeeding.

+ They tell all pregnant mothers why and how to breastfeed.

+ They help you start breastfeeding within one hour after your baby is born.

+ They show you how to breastfeed, and they show you how to keep your milk coming in even if you have to be away from your baby for work or other reasons.

+ They support the finding that newborns should be fed only breast milk.

+ They encourage you and the baby to stay together all day and all night (called *rooming in*).

+ They encourage you to feed your baby whenever she wants to nurse rather than at certain times.

+ They do not give pacifiers to breastfed babies.

+ They encourage you to join a group of mothers who breastfeed. They tell you how to contact a group near you.

+ They have a written policy about breastfeeding. All the employees know about and use the ideas in the policy.

+ They teach their employees the skills they need to carry out these steps.

Take all the information you have learned in this chapter with you when you are interviewing medical personnel. Also, don't hesitate to contact the nurse manager in the labor and delivery department of your local hospital and question her. Show this chapter to your doula—she may be able to help with some of your questions because of her own experiences in the hospitals she has worked in.

Back Matter

♦

Appendix I
Books to Read and Read Again

"The essence of knowledge is, having it, to apply it;
not having it, to confess your ignorance."
    —Confucius

Hundreds of books are available to help prepare you for your special day. There are books about everything from getting pregnant to putting your kids through college—and everything in between! These are some of my favorites about the childbearing years.

Pregnancy and Childbirth

Brewer, Gail Sforza and Tom Brewer, *What Every Pregnant Woman Should Know*, Random House (September 1977) ASIN 039441117X

England, Pam and Rob Horowitz, *Birthing From Within: An Extraordinary Guide to Childbirth Preparation*, Partera (July 1998) ISBN 0965987302

Gaskin, Ina May, *Ina May's Guide to Childbirth*, Bantam (March 2003) ISBN 0553381156

Jimenez, Sherry, *The Pregnant Woman's Comfort Guide,* Avery Penguin Putnam (April 1992) ASIN 0895294907

Kitzinger, Sheila, *The Complete Book of Pregnancy and Childbirth,* Knopf (December 2003) ISBN 0375710477

Kitzinger, Sheila, *The Experience of Childbirth,* Penguin (July 1984) ASIN 014022548X

McCutcheon, Susan, *Natural Childbirth the Bradley Way, Revised,* Plume (July 1996) ISBN 0452276594

Peterson, Gayle, *An Easier Childbirth: A Mother's Guide for Birthing Normally,* J. P. Tarcher (November 1991) ASIN 0874776651

Simkin, Penny, Janet Whalley, and Ann Keppler, *Pregnancy, Childbirth, and the Newborn: The Complete Guide,* Meadowbrook (August 2001) ISBN 074321241X

Simkin, Penny and Ruth Ancheta, *The Labor Progress Handbook: Early Interventions to Prevent and Treat Dystocia,* Blackwell Science (March 2000) ISBN 0632052813

Birthing Choices

Arms, Suzanne, *Immaculate Deception II: Myth, Magic & Birth,* Celestial Arts (September 1994) ISBN 0890876339

Davis, Elizabeth, *Heart and Hands: A Midwife's Guide to Pregnancy and Birth,* Celestial Arts (December 1997) ISBN 0890878382

Davis-Floyd, Robbie, *Birth as an American Rite of Passage,* University of California Press (September 1993) ISBN 0520084314

Davis-Floyd, Robbie and Carolyn Sargent, eds., *Childbirth and Authoritative Knowledge,* University of California Press (July 1997) ISBN 0520207858

Gaskin, Ina May, *Spiritual Midwifery,* Book Pub (April 2002) ISBN 1570671044

Goer, Henci, *The Thinking Woman's Guide to a Better Birth,* Perigee (October 1999) ISBN 0399525173

Harper, Barbara and Suzanne Arms (photographer), *Gentle Birth Choices: A Guide to Making Informed Decisions about Birthing Centers, Birth Attendants, Water Birth, Home Birth, Hospital Birth,* Inner Traditions (May 1994) ISBN 0892814802

Kitzinger, Sheila, *Homebirth,* DK Publishing (September 1991) ASIN 1879431017

Kitzinger, Sheila, *Your Baby Your Way, Making Pregnancy Decisions and Birth Plans,* Pantheon Books (June 1987) ASIN 0394545737

Leboyer, Frederick, *Birth Without Violence: Revised Edition of the Classic,* Inner Traditions (May 2002) ISBN 0892819839

Mauger, Benig, *Reclaiming the Spirituality of Birth: Healing for Mothers and Babies,* Healing Arts (March 2000) ISBN 0892818964

Odent, Michel, *Birth Reborn,* Birth Works (September 1994) ISBN 0964203693

Odent, Michel, *Primal Health: Understanding the Critical Period between Conception and the First Birthday,* Clairview Books (October 2002) ISBN 1902636333

Simkin, Penny, *The Birth Partner: Second Edition,* Harvard Common (June 2001) ISBN 1558321950

Wickham, Sara, *What's Right for Me?* AIMS (2002)

Doulas

Klaus, Marshall, MD, John Kennel, and Phyllis Klaus, *The Doula Book: How a Trained Labor Companion Can Help You Have a Shorter, Easier, and Healthier Birth,* Perseus (November 2002) ISBN 0738206091

Perez, Paulina, *Doula Programs,* Cutting Edge (April 1998) ISBN 0964115972

Breastfeeding

Eiger, Marvin S., Sally Wendkos Olds, *The Complete Book of Breastfeeding: Revised,* Bantam (September 1999) ISBN 0553580744

Gotsch, Gwen, Anwar Fazal, and July Torgus, *The Womanly Art of Breastfeeding,* Plume (September 1997) ISBN 0452279089

Huggins, Kathleen, *The Nursing Mother's Companion,* National Book Network (July 1999) ISBN 1558321527

Kitzinger, Sheila, *The Experience of Breastfeeding,* Penguin USA (December 1990) ASIN 0140093524

Tamaro, Janet, *So That's What They're For! Breastfeeding Basics,* Adams Media (March 1998) ISBN 1580620418

Vaginal Birth After Cesarean and Cesarean Birth

Cohen, Nancy and Lois J. Estner, *Silent Knife: Cesarean Prevention and Vaginal Birth after Cesarean,* Bergin & Garvey (March 1983) ISBN 0897890272

Crawford, Karis and Johanne Walters, *Natural Childbirth After Cesarean: A Practical Guide,* Blackwell Science (January 1996) ASIN 086542490X

Jones, Carl, *The Expectant Parent's Guide to Preventing a Cesarean Section,* Bergin & Garvey (March 1991) ISBN 0897892232

Korte, Diana, *A Good Birth, A Safe Birth: Choosing and Having the Childbirth Experience You Want,* Harvard Common (December 1992) ISBN 1558320423

Korte, Diana, *The VBAC Companion,* Harvard Common (January 1998) ISBN 1558321292

Madsen, Lynn, *Rebounding From Childbirth,* Bergin & Garvey (July 1994) ISBN 0897893484

Panuthos, Claudia, *Ended Beginnings,* Greenwood (November 1990) ISBN 089789054X

Herbs in Pregnancy and Childbirth

Fetrow, Charles W. and Juan R. Avila, *The Complete Guide to Herbal Medicines,* Springhouse (January 2000) ISBN 158255062X

Gardner-Goodson, Joy, *Healing Yourself During Pregnancy,* Crossing Press (June 2000) ASIN 0895942518

Gladstar, Rosemary, *Herbal Healing for Women,* Fireside (November 1993) ISBN 0671767674

Lust, John, *The Herb Book,* Benedict Lust Publications (June 2001) ISBN 0879040556

McIntyre, Anne, *The Complete Woman's Herbal: A Manual of Healing Herbs and Nutrition for Personal Well-Being and Family Care,* Henry Holt & Co. (January 1995) ASIN 0805035370

Weed, Susun S., *Wise Woman's Herbal for the Childbearing Years,* Ash Tree (June 1985) ISBN 0961462000

HypnoBirthing® and Hypnosis

Mongan, Marie F., *HypnoBirthing: A Celebration of Life,* Rivertree (April 1996) ISBN 0966351711

O'Neill, Michelle Leclaire, *Creative Childbirth: The Leclaire Method of Easy Birthing Through Hypnosis and Rational-Intuitive Thought,* Papyrus (March 1993) ISBN 0963308734

Yoga and Prenatal Exercise

Berg, Vibeke, *Yoga During Pregnancy,* Simon & Shuster (March 1983) ASIN 0671459872

Hoare, Sophy, *Yoga and Pregnancy,* Unwin Hyman (October 1986) ASIN 0041490614

Noble, Elizabeth, *Essential Exercises for the Childbearing year: A Guide to Health and Comfort before and after Your Baby is Born,* New Life Images (September 2003) ISBN 0964118319

Olkin, Sylvia Klein, *Positive Pregnancy Fitness: A Guide to a More Comfortable Pregnancy and Easier Birth through Exercise and Relaxation,* Avery Penguin Putnam (March 1992) ASIN 0895294818

Simkin, Diana, *The Complete Pregnancy Exercise Program,* Plume (May 1982) ASIN 0452254175

Trivell, Lisa, *I Can't Believe It's Yoga For Pregnancy and After,* Hatherleigh (August 2000) ISBN 1578260469

Reflexology and Acupressure

Enzer, Suzanne, *Maternity Reflexology,* Soul to Sole Reflexology (2003) ISBN 0646313924

Enzer, Suzanne, *Reflexology: A Tool for Midwives,* Soul to Sole Reflexology (July 2000) ISBN 0957721501

Gach, Michael Reed, *Acupressure's Potent Points,* Bantam (November 1990) ISBN 0553349708

Teeguarden, Iona Marsaa, *The Joy of Feeling: Bodymind Acupressure,* Japan Publications (July 1989) ISBN 0870406345

Touch and Massage

Montagu, Ashley, *Touching: The Human Significance of the Skin,* Perennial
(September 1986) ISBN 0060960280

Appendix II
Websites to Surf

"It's the friends that you can call up at 4am that matter."
—Marlene Dietrich

Thank you Steve Jobs and Bill Gates for access to the world. Here are some great sites to explore and enjoy, which will lead you to other sites and on and on.

Doula Sites

birthmarket.com

- ✦ Midwifery Today's Directory of Products and Services.
- ✦ Includes "Find a Midwife" and "Find a Doula."

birthpartners.com

- ✦ Helping to find natural childbirth choices.

Specialties include:

- ✦ Birth & Pregnancy Art
- ✦ Birth Doulas
- ✦ Birth Photographers

- ✦ Breastfeeding Support
- ✦ Childbirth Educators
- ✦ Chiropractors
- ✦ Holistic Doctors
- ✦ HypnoBirthing
- ✦ Massage Therapists
- ✦ Midwives
- ✦ Postpartum Doulas
- ✦ Pregnancy Photographers
- ✦ Pregnancy Yoga
- ✦ Psychotherapists

dona.com

DONA is the acronym for Doulas of North America, an international association of doulas who are trained to provide the highest quality emotional, physical, and educational support to women and their families during childbirth and postpartum. DONA is the premier doula organization founded by Marshall Klaus MD, Phyllis Klaus, John Kennell MD, Penny Simkin, and Annie Kennedy in 1992. Evidence-based certification programs are offered for both birth doulas and postpartum doulas.

Membership in DONA includes over 4,700 birth and postpartum doulas.

This website was created to aid in searching for and securing a doula for your birth. Most of the doulas in this book were certified through DONA.

idoula.com

This site is dedicated to helping birthing and new families make the important decisions that come along with new parenthood. Their second priority is supporting new doulas that also have decisions to make and paths to choose. The role of a doula is to provide support for the birthing and new mother.

Recommended reading for birth doulas: www.motherstuff.com, a mega-index of mother-knowledge on the Internet. Covers birth, breastfeeding, midwifery, parenting, preemies, health, and pregnancy. (Doula links are mainly for the actual doula.)

pals-doulas.org

The Pacific Association for Labor Support (PALS) is a membership organization that promotes, develops, and supports doulas and the doula profession. The primary mission of the doula profession is to positively impact the childbearing experience for women and their families.

pregnacy.about.com

This is a pregnancy search engine. When you enter this site you will find a search space. Enter the information that you want and it'll take you there. About pregnancy and birth. Lots of links to other sites.

my.webmd.com

Another great search engine for childbirth, pregnancy, breastfeeding, and finding doulas. In the search box type "Much Ado About Doulas." This is a good site.

Organization Sites

bradleybirth.com

This is the site of the American Academy of Husband-Coached Childbirth.

This organization shows fathers to not only be there for their wives during labor and their baby's birth but to be able to help their partner effectively breathe and relax during her contractions. Good site to involve your husband in your birth.

cappa.net

CAPPA (Childbirth and Postpartum Professional Association) is an international organization that was founded in 1998 to offer the highest level of professional membership and training to childbirth educators, lactation educators, labor doulas, antepartum doulas, and postpartum doulas.

Training and certifying labor and postpartum doula and childbirth educators.

ican-online.org

The International Cesarean Awareness Network, Inc. (ICAN) is a nonprofit organization founded by Esther Booth Zorn in 1982. ICAN's mission is to prevent unnecessary cesareans through education, to provide support for cesarean recovery, and to promote VBAC. Their job is educating women to help prevent the need for cesareans. Offers newsletters, conferences and nationwide support groups

vbac.com

This website provides childbearing women and maternity care professionals access to research-based information, resources, continuing education, and support for VBAC (vaginal birth after cesarean). A great site to answer questions about avoiding another cesarean on the next birth.

icea.org

ICEA (International Childbirth Education Association) offers outstanding professional certification programs, professional training workshops, an annual international convention, and numerous publications to assist the educator in her own development as well as for the enhancement of educational programs for expectant and new parents.

lamaze-childbirth.com

Lamaze International was created to promote, support, and protect natural birth through education and advocacy. Lamaze International believes that women who are fully informed, confident, and supported will want normal birth.

Lamaze class homepage: This site will direct you, after informing you about them, on how to find a Lamaze instructor in your area. These are good people wanting you to have a sensational birth.

mana.org

Midwives Alliance of North America (MANA) was created to provide a nurturing forum for support and cooperation among midwives. Through their collective strength, they can ensure midwifery care for all mothers and their babies throughout North America. They can provide you with information on midwifery and referrals to midwives in your area.

midwiferytoday.com

The heart and science of birth. Excellent website and information source. A website you can spend hours on. They have information for mothers, parents to be, midwives, doulas, prenatal instructors, and all forms of birthing advocates. They advertise and give conferences all over the world to further the education of men and women interested in the birthing process. They have numerous publications you can buy, a great magazine you can subscribe to, online newsletters, and much, much more to explore.

motherfriendly.org

CIMS (Coalition for Improving Maternity Services) was created to promote a wellness model of maternity care that will improve birth outcomes and substantially reduce costs. I believe this organization will change how women are treated during their labor and the birth of their baby in hospitals.

Breastfeeding Sites

lalecheleague.org

La Leche League believes that mothering through breastfeeding is the most natural and effective way of understanding and satisfying the needs of the baby. Their website gives you a lot of information on how to understand and find the right person to help you be successful in breastfeeding. They are also wrote *The Womanly Art of Breastfeeding*, a big "must buy." Best breastfeeding help around. You can call them 9am-3pm CST at 1-800-LA-LECHE.

famsupport.com

A site for Breastfeeding accessories. They offer expectant and new mothers the highest quality Medela® breast pumps, nursing bras, breastfeeding supplies, and lactation services. They specialize in making motherhood easier by offering you a full line of breastfeeding products and services.

breastfeeding.com

This is another website that you can click on for hundreds of helpful pieces of information about breastfeeding support and reading material, help for working moms, and other information for the breastfeeding family.

breastfeeding.co.uk

British breastfeeding and childbirth resource. Somewhat like the previous site.

moonlily.com/breastfeed

Exploring Inner and Outer Dimensions. Kind of a weird website, but some good information.

HypnoBirthing® Sites

hypnobirthing.com

HypnoBirthing is a unique method of relaxed, natural childbirth education, enhanced by hypnosis techniques, providing the missing link that allows women to use their natural instincts to bring about a safer, easier, more comfortable birthing in a way that most mirrors nature. Emphasis is placed on both pregnancy and childbirth as well as on HypnoBirthing. Official site of HypnoBirthing.

hypnobirthingnorthwest.com

This sites helps you find classes and tells you more about HypnoBirthing. Speaks for itself.

hometown.aol.com/doulatracy/index

Birth empowerment support team.

expage.com/page/hypnosislinks

This is a links site to all types of hypnosis and HypnoBirthing web sites all around the states and in the UK.

Childbirth Class Sites

birthworks.org

Birth Works® embodies the philosophy of developing a woman's self confidence, and trust and faith in her ability to give birth. It is the goal of their childbirth classes and doula services as well as their childbirth educator and doula certification programs to promote safe and loving birth experiences through education, introspection, and confident action.

Classes, doula services, educators.

babycenter.com

Birthright is about:

+ Offering accessible and affordable quality childbirth products, services, and education

+ Providing women with the proper tools and information to make informed choices in alliance with a safe and healthy labor experience

+ Promoting advocacy on behalf of women and their unborn babies

+ Encouraging women to pursue their ideal birth experience

+ Offering accessible and affordable quality

lamazevideo.com

You can purchase Lamaze videos to view at home and watch over and over again. Great idea for those can't get to a class but still want the information the classes offer.

Pregnancy and Baby Sites

babyzone.com

Information from preconception to parenting. Fun site, lots of information. Tons of pregnancy and baby stuff.

childbirth.org

Pregnancy is a very special time in a person's life. Educating yourselves to be good consumers, knowing your options, and how to provide yourselves with the best possible care are essential to a healthy pregnancy. Enjoy the many links of an educational, informational, and personal nature. Great baby center.

firstbabymall.com

Just what it says: a first baby mall great shopping for all kinds of pregnancy and baby stuff. Products, classes, and resources.

ivillage.com

At this site you can explore everything from babies, horoscopes, and health and diet to entertainment, food and parenting, and much more. Fun site to explore anything about women's health.

parentsplace.com

Supported by ivillage.com. There are tons of things to explore. Covers fertility, infertility, twins, baby, health, pregnancy loss, newborn, and lots more.

parentsplace.com/pregnancy/calendar

The Interactive Pregnancy Calendar will build a day-by-day customized calendar detailing the development of a baby from before conception to birth. Create a calendar to see your baby progress.

pregnancydaily.com

The Pregnancy Daily will tell you how pregnant you are in days and weeks, how many days left until D-day, and the baby's gestational age in days and weeks. And every day there's something more. Another great calendar site.

pregnancyguideonline.com

For each of the forty weeks of pregnancy, you'll find information about baby's development, the types of changes that occur within mom's pregnant body, tidbits for dads, specific info for pregnant moms of multiples, inspirational thoughts, and suggested reading. This has a fun place to track your pregnancy week by week.

pregnancytoday.com

The journal for parents-to-be. From pre-conception to parenting and everything in between.

Midwifery and Homebirths

rslnetwork.com/midwifery/homebirths.html

This has tons of homebirth websites and information to explore.

pasterik.homestead.com/homebirth.html

The website is provided for those who are interested in or are planning a homebirth. Interesting stories and pictures. Some are pretty graphic but all are so exciting. A homebirth website. Nice stories and pictures.

midwiferytoday.com/articles/homebirthchoice.asp

An article from Jill Cohen and Marti Dorsey on a homebirth choice. This will also lead you to their home page that is full of information.

Herbs in Pregnancy, Childbirth, and Postpartum

www.gardenguides.com/herbs/preg.htm

This is where you can find lots of information on herbs and how they are useful in pregnancy and after. This also gives you an idea of which herbs not to take during your pregnancy.

geocities.com/HotSprings/5316/pregnancy.html

Herbs that are useful in pregnancy. Not a lot of information, but useful.

sbherbals.com/UsefulInPregnancy.html

Another site that gives you information on herbal use during your pregnancy and after. Some links at the bottom of the page to lead you into further study.

gentlebirth.org/archives/herbs.html

A link from gentlebirth.org that will give you herbal information.

http://moonlily.com/herb/default.htm

This is another page from moonlily.com that is fun to play with and explore.

http://pregnancytoday.com/reference/articles/ herbspreg.htm

Part of PregnancyToday.com's website. Informative; links to other sites.

Yoga

about.com

In search, type "yoga." Lists at the bottom of the page show yoga sites. This is a great pregnancy/birth site with good subject lists from which to choose.

yoga.com

In the bottom left-hand section there is a linked called "Why Pregnancy Yoga?"—a good article. Also, there is a lot of information about Yoga in general.

If you view the index you will find a section "For Prenatal and Postnatal Resources."

socalbirth.org/shelly/yoga.htm

This site has yoga exercises that are specifically tailored for strengthening and relaxing the rapidly changing body of a pregnant woman. These simple exercises, combined with learned breathing techniques, will guide the pregnant woman through pregnancy and labor. Nice easy graphics to follow and a good start in learning more about yoga.

healthandyoga.com/html/preg.html

Explore this to find something that will help you learn more about breathing and relaxation through yoga.

healthandyoga.com/html/pyogaex.html

Nice site. Lots of information, and they have (on their side panel) a Pregnancy Plan using yoga to take you through your trimesters.

Hey! Who's Having This Baby Anyway?

HeyAnyway.com

The home website for this book and its author.

EndTableBooks.com/HeyAnyway

Where you can order additional copies of *Hey!*, or copies in quantity.

Appendix III
Contributors

"A master can tell you what he expects of you.
A teacher, though, awakens your own experiences."
—Patricia Neal

As I compiled this book, various birth professionals and organizations granted me permission to use their materials in order to give readers a well-rounded presentation. I can't thank these women enough for so willingly sharing their time, energy, and insight with us. It is gratifying to know that so many people care enough to share their skills with others.*

The list that follows organizes these contributors' names by the state or country in which they live. I hope it will help you locate a professional near you.

And as of this writing, my email address is Breck@writeme.com. Please feel free to write to me!

Arizona

Lynn Davies
Mesa, Arizona

Rosie Ruiz, doula
Phoenix, Arizona

Greta Sprenkeling
Scottsdale, Arizona

Arkansas

Ann J. Johnson,
BS, ICCE, BE, CD (DONA)
Bentonville, Arkansas

California

Gina Acosta, ICCE, CD (DONA)
Special Deliveries by Gina
Canyon Country, California

Jeannine Z. Albertine, CMT, doula
Agourea Hills, California

Judy Ballinger, RN, CMT, CD
Birth & Bonding
Albany, California

Tara Beasley
San Francisco, California

Sabrina Cuddy, MPH, CD (DONA)
Redwood City, California

Chantal DeSoto,
certified clinical hypnotherapist,
doula.
Advanced Health Resources,
Santa Cruz, California

Glenda Hamilton,
postpartum doula.
San Francisco, California

Laine Holman
Santa Rosa, California

Kim Killackey
Covena Baldwin Park, California

Meghan Lewis, PhD, CMT
Berkeley, California

Kris Luitwieler CLE, CD
Redlands, California

Sarah McKay, doula
Elk Grove, California

Kathleen Magee, doula
Rancho Palo Verdes, California

Rosemary Mason, CCE, birth/
postpartum doula
North County Doulas
San Diego, California

Sue O'Connor, BA, CPM, former
CAM chairwoman
Los Osos, California

Sabine Omvik, CD (DONA),
childbirth educator (Birthing From
Within), nursing-mother
counselor, mother of two
Scotts Valley, California

Jennifer Perry, professional
childbirth assistant/doula, fertility
consultant. "Empowering Women,
Changing Our World"
Sacramento, California

Felicia Roche CD (DONA)
Berkeley, California

Maryanne Savino, birth doula
Oakland, California

Connie Sultana, ICCE, CD
(DONA) Rohnert Park, California

Juliana Walker,
B.A. in biology, doula.
San Rafael, California

Giselle Whitwell, RMT, doula
Center for Prenatal Music
Los Angeles, California

Holly Wiersma, CD (DONA)
Walnut Creek, California

Colorado

Anne DeMaria, CD, LCCE, CIMI
Edubirth Childbirth Services
Fort Collins, Colorado

Florida

Ramona Majewski, CD
Blessed Miracles Doula Service
Fort Myers and Naples, Florida

Cindy Morris, CD (DONA)
DONA Florida state representative
Treasures at Birth
professional labor support
provider. Doula service & birth
ball distributor.
Sarasota, Florida

Fran Slafky, CD, ICCE
New Port Richey, Florida

Susan Woodhouse
South Florida

Idaho

Jennifer Schepper,
CD (DONA), CPM
Kuna, Idaho

Illinois

Julie Reams, CD (DONA)
Illinois

Ellen Richter, CD (DONA)
Cary, Illinois

Indiana

Becca Cartledge, RN, BSN
Indianapolis, Indiana

Donna Marcosson, birth doula,
MOA. Muncie, Indiana

Kansas

Teri Bavley
Prairie Village, Kansas

Maryland

Brenda Lane, ICCE, CE
Arnold, Maryland

Gwen Peters, CD (DONA),
AAHCC, ICEA
Columbia, Maryland

Georgeanne Saddington
Aberdeen, Maryland

Massachusetts

Dena Carmosino, doula,
HypnoBirthing instructor,
apprentice midwife
"Birthsong"
Acton, Massachusetts

Laura Sevika Douglass,
yoga instructor
Watertown, Massachusetts

Michigan

Linda Sheppard,
RN, ICCE, CD, LC
Harbor Springs, Michigan

Missouri

Sr. Gladys Leigh, Congregation of
St. Joseph
CD (DONA), massage therapist
and infant massage instructor
St. Louis, Missouri

Gloria Squitiro, CD, CBE
(AAHCC)
Owner of Birthways
Kansas City, Missouri

New Jersey

Heather Bella
Labor of Love Pregnancy Support
Heart and Hands Doula Training
Program
Passaic, North Jersey

Augustine Daniels, CBE
New Jersey

Debra Pascali-Bonaro, CD
(DONA), CPD, CAPPA, CBE
CIMS fundraising chairperson
doula program design and
consultation
president, Mother Love, Inc.
River Vale, New Jersey

New York

Bonu deCaires, CD (DONA)
New York, New York

Alice Gilgoff, LM
Owner, Postpartum Services
New York

Robin Goodwin-Millap, CD
New York, New York

Lynne Howard, CD (DONA)
Walworth, New York

Tammie Moberg, CD (DONA),
CCE (CAPPA)
Pine City, New York

Barbara O'Brien, RN, CBE
Staten Island, New York

Kathleen Ruggio. LPN, CD, HBCE
Oswego, New York

Shanti Sunshine Volpe, RN, BSN,
CIMI, CD, CDD, CYT
Long Island, New York

North Carolina

Pat Steimer, RN
Fayetteville, North Carolina

Angel Turlington, RN, CD
Henderson, North Carolina

Ohio

Pam Udy, ICAN Ed. Dir., Utah
chapter leader
Celebrating the Gift of Birth
Cleveland, Ohio

Oklahoma

Donna Leach, MS Ed, CD (DONA)
Broken Arrow/Tulsa, Oklahoma

Oregon

Kelly Townsend, president,
Doulas of Southern Oregon
Medford, Oregon

Pennsylvania

Julie Thompson, CD (DONA)
Sugar Grove, Pennsylvania

South Carolina

Allison Erwin
Honea Path, South Carolina

Linda Weaver
Spartanburg. South Carolina

South Dakota

Angela Rabenberg, CD (DONA)
Gentle Birth Doula Services
Brookings, South Dakota

Texas

Linda Cameron,
CD (DONA) CBE (CAPPA)
breastfeeding educator
Henrietta, Texas

Lanell Coultas, CD (DONA)
Texas DONA state representative

Myra Lowrie, BS, ICCE, IBCLC,
CD (DONA)
Sugar Land, Texas

Lori Wiseheart,
RMT, CD (DONA) CBE, MTI
Waco, Texas

Utah

Tara Tulley CPM
Payson, Utah

Virginia

Avery E. Morgan, RN, BSN
Virginia

Washington

Blue Bradley
Twisp, Washington

Shellie Moore
Langley, Whidbey Island,
Washington

Andrea Nesheim, doula
Seattle, Washington

Patti Ramos Photography
pregnancy, birth, newborn,
and family
Tacoma, Washington

Heather Shelley, CCCE, doula,
bellycasts, photography
CAPPA Washington state
representative
Bellevue, Washington

West Virginia

Kari Shelton CDDNA
Martainsburg, West Virginia

Wisconsin

Karen Kohls,
CD (DONA), PT, CCE
Middleton, Wisconsin

Alberta, Canada

Deb the Doula MacFarlane
Calgary, Alberta

Elaine Montgomery
Calgary, Alberta

Kathy Montgomery, CD
Calgary, Alberta

British Columbia, Canada

Linda Baril, reflexologist/
instructor (RAC), CD (DONA),
prenatal instructor (ICEA), doula
trainer (DONA)
Comox, Vancouver Island, British
Columbia

Lisa Bognar
Comox Valley, Vancouver Island,
British Columbia

*Prince Edward Island,
Canada*

Michelle Prouse, doula
Charlottetown, Prince Edward
Island, Canada

Mexico

Guadalupe Trueba, CD (DONA);
CBE, Mexican Society for
Psychoprophylaxis in Obstetrics;
perinatal educator;
Lamaze childbirth educator
Mexico City, Mexico

Appendix IV

Abbreviation Key

"Whatever women do they must do twice as well as men to be thought half as good. Luckily, this is not difficult."
    —Charlotte Whitton

AAHCC: American Association of Health Care Consultants
ACHI: Association for Childbirth at Home, Intl.
ACOG: American College of Obstetricians and Gynecologists
BSN: Bachelor of Science in Nursing
CAPPA: Childbirth and Postpartum Professional Association
CBE: ChildBirth Educator
CD: Certified Doula
CDC: Center for Disease Control
CIMS: Coalition for Improving Maternity Services
CMT: Certified Massage Therapist
CNM: Certified Nurse Midwife
CPM: Certified Professional Midwife
DEM: Direct Entry Midwife
DONA: Doulas of North America
HBCE: HypnoBirth Certified Educator
IBCLC: International Board Certified Lactation Consultant
ICAN: International Cesarean Awareness Network
ICEA: International Childbirth Education Association
LDM: Licensed Direct-Entry Midwife
LM: Licensed Midwife
MANA: Midwives Alliance of North America
MTI: Mission Training Institute
NICU: Neonatal Intensive Care Unit
NIH: National Institute of Health
PALS: Pacific Association for Labor Support
UNICEF: United Nations International Children's Emergency Fund
VBAC: Vaginal Birth After Cesarean
WHO: World Health Organization

Note: *HypnoBirthing* is a registered trademark of owner and founder Marie Mongan of the HypnoBirthing Institute[SM] in Epsom, NH. *Astroglide, Medela,* and *Birth Works* are registered trademarks.

Endnotes

Introduction

1. M. Klaus, et al., "Effects of social support during parturition on maternal and infant morbidity," *British Medical Journal*, Vol. 293, pp. 585–587, 1986

2. J. Kennel, "Medical intervention: The effect of social support during labor," *Pediatric Res.*, Vol. 23, p. 211A, 1988

3. E. Hemmiki, "A trial of continuous human support during labor: Feasibility, interventions and mother's satisfaction," *Journal of Psychosomatic Obstetrics and Gynecology,* Vol. 11, pp. 239–250, 1990

4. M. Wagner, *Pursuing the Birth Machine,* ACE Graphics, Camperdown, Australia, 1994

Chapter 2 — *Hiring the Help*

1. Information adapted from *Ultrasound? Unsound,* by Jean Robinson and Beverley Lawrence Beech. Robinson and Beech reveal the hazards of repeated use of ultrasound during pregnancy, including miscarriage, premature labor, and false diagnosis of placental previa and of growth retardation, both of which can result in unnecessary C-section.

2. Pat Sonnernstuhl, "Midwifery in the United States," Feb. 11, 1998. Archive—name: medicine/midwifery/united-states.

3. L.E. Mehl, G.H. Peterson, M. Whitt and W.H. Hawes, "Outcomes of Elective Home Births, A Series of 1,146 Cases," *Journal of Reproductive Medicine* 19: 1997, pp. 281–9.

Chapter 3 — *Medications in Labor*

1. http://www.manbit.com

2. http://dacc.bsd.uchicago.edu

3. P. England, CNM, MA; R. Howowitz, PhD; *Birthing From Within,* Paterna Press, 1998, p. 248.

4. http://dacc.bsd.uchicago.edu

5. http://sblomberg.com/epidural/

6. http://sblomberg.com/epidural/

7. http://sblomberg.com/epidural/

8. http://www.manbit.com/oa/c84.htm

9. http://dacc.bsd.uchicago.edu

10. http://cardiology.medscape.com

11. http://www.epidural.net

12. http://www.csen.com/anesthesia/book/#ch11

13. http://www.healing-arts.org

14. http://www.pregnancy.about.com

15. www.gentlebirth.org

16. http://www.gentlebirth.org

17. Goer, Henci, *The Thinking Woman's Guide to a Better Birth*, Berkley Publishing Group, 1999, p. 133.

18. ibid., p. 270.

19. ibid., pp. 270–271.

20. http://www.ncbi.nlm.nih.gov

21. H. Goer, *The Thinking Woman's Guide to a Better Birth*, pp. 270–271.

22. http://www.ncbi.nlm.nih.gov

23. H. Goer, *Obstetric Myth Versus Research Realities*, Bergin & Garvey, 1995, p. 254.

24. http://www.phypc.med.wayne.edu/jfp/jc0595b

25. http://www.soap.org

26. H. Goer, *The Thinking Woman's Guide to a Better Birth*, p. 265.

27. http://www.phypc.med.wayne.edu/jfp/jc0595b.htm

28. H. Goer, *The Thinking Woman's Guide to a Better Birth*, p. 266.

29. Pam England, CNM, MA; Rob Horowitz, PhD; *Birthing From Within*, p. 248.

30. H. Goer, *The Thinking Woman's Guide to a Better Birth*, p. 157.

31. ibid., p. 249.

32. H. Goer, *The Thinking Woman's Guide to a Better Birth*, p. 157.

33. ibid, p. 249.

34. James Nelison, et al., *A Guide to Effective Care in Pregnancy and Childbirth*, Oxford University Press, 1985

Chapter 7 — *Homebirth*

1. Dr. Lewis Mehl, "Home Birth versus Hospital Birth: Comparisons of Outcomes of Matched Populations," presented on October 20, 1976, before the 104th annual meeting of the American Public Health Association. For further information contact the Institute for Childbirth and Family Research, 2522 Dana St., Suite 201, Berkeley, CA 94704. *www.healing-arts.org/mehl-madrona*

2. *Texas Lay Midwifery Program, Six-Year Report, 1983–1989,* Berstein & Bryant, Appendix VIIIf, Texas Department of Health, 1100 West 49th St., Austin, TX 78756-3199. You can check out their website at *www.midwife-cpm.com/DWIsItSafe.htm*

3. Madrona, Lewis & Morgaine, "The Future of Midwifery in the United States," NAPSAC News, Fall-Winter, 1993, p. 30

Chapter 8 — *Waterbirths*

1. Paul Johnson, "Birth under water—to breathe or not to breathe," *British Journal of Obstetrics and Gynecology*, Vol. 103, 1996, pp. 202–208

2. J.E. Fewell, P. Johnson, "Upper airway dynamics during breathing and during apnea in fetal lambs," *Journal of Physiology,* Vol. 339, 1983, pp. 495–504

3. R. Harding, P. Johnson, M. McClelland, "Liquid sensitive laryngeal receptors in the developing sheep, cat, and monkey," *Journal of Physiology*, Vol. 277, 1978, pp. 409–422

4. P. Karlberg, et al., "Alteration of the infant's thorax during vaginal delivery," *Acta Obstetrica Gynecol Scandavia.* Vol. 41, 1987, p. 223

5. R. Gilbert, P. Tookey, "Perinatal mortality and morbidity among babies delivered in water: surveillance study and postal survey," *British Medical Journal* Vol. 39, 21 August 1999, pp. 483–487

6. Personal interviews with Barbara Harper, 1989

7. M. Rosenthal, "Warm-water immersion in labor and birth," *Female Patient,* Vol. 16, August 1991, pp. 44–51

8. D. Garland, K. Jones, "Waterbirth: updating the evidence," *British Journal of Midwifery*, Vol. 5, No 6, June 1997, pp. 368–373

9. M. Eriksson, L. Ladfors, L. Mattson, et al., "Warm tub bath during labor. A study of 1385 women with prelabor rupture of the membranes after 34 weeks of gestation," *Acta Obstetricia et Gynecologieca Scandinavica*, Vol. 75, No. 7, August 1996, pp. 642–644

10. D. Garland, K. Jones, "Waterbirth: updating the evidence," *British Journal of Midwifery*, June, Vol. 5, No. 6, June 1997, pp. 368–373

11. P. Siegel, "Does bath water enter the vagina?" *Journal of Obstetrics and Gynecology*, Vol. 15, 1960, pp. 660–661

12. J. Rush, S. Burlock, K. Lambert, et al., "The effects of whirlpool baths in labor: a randomized, controlled trial," *Birth*, September, Vol. 23, No. 3, Sept. 1996, pp. 136–143

13. Personal communication with Polly Malby, CMN, 1999

14. L. Brown, "The tide of waterbirth has turned: audit of water birth," *British Jounal of Midwifery*, Vol. 6, No. 4, April 1998, pp. 236–243

15. M. Favero, "Risk of AIDS and other STDs from swimming pools and whirlpools is nil," *Postgraduate Medicine*, Vol. 80, No. 1, 1986, p. 283

16. Global Maternal/Child Health Association, "Procedures and Protocols for warm water immersion in labor and birth," 1996, revised Jan 2000

17. Personal correspondence, Lynn Springer, RNC, 2000

18. F. Hadad, "Labor and birth in water: an obstetrician's observations over a decade," *Waterbirth Unplugged*, BFM Press, London, 1996, pp. 96–108

19. V. Katz, R. Ryder, R. Cefalo, S. Carmichael, R. Goolsby, "A comparison of bed rest and immersion for treating the edema of pregnancy," *Obstetrics and Gynecology*, Vol. 75, No. 2, Feb 1990, pp. 147–151

20. M. Odent, "Use of water during labor—updated recommendations," MIDIRS, Vol. 8, No. 1, March 1998, pp. 68–69

21. D. Garland, *Waterbirth—An Attitude to Care*, Books for Midwives Press, London, 1995, revised 2000, p. 23

22. E. Burn, K. Greenish, "Pooling information," *Nursing Times*, Vol. 89, No. 8, 1993, pp. 47–49

23. D. Garland, K. Jone, "Waterbirth: updating the evidence," *British Journal of Midwifery*, Vol. 5, No. 6, June 1997, p. 371

24. H. Ponette, "Water births: My experience of 1600 waterbirths, including breeches and twins," Abstract published for the World Waterbirth Conference, Wimbly Hall, London, England, 1995

25. Waterbirth International Practitioner Survey report, 2000—unpublished

26. Suzanna Napierala, *Waterbirth: A Midwife's Perspective*, Bergin and Garvey, New York, 1994

27. Department of Health, Changing Childbirth Report of the Expert Maternity Group (The Cumberledge Report), London, 1993, HMSO

28. United Kingdom Central Council for Nursing, Midwifery and Health Visiting, Registrar's Letter—Position Statement on Waterbirth, April 1994

Chapter 9 — *Birth Plans*

1. Leah Albers and C. J. Krulewitch, "Electronic Fetal Monitoring in the United States in the 1980s," *Obstetrics & Gynecology*, 82:8–10, 1993

2. *pregnancy.about.com/library/weekly/aa070797.htm*

3. J.N. Robinson et al., "Predictors of Episiotomy at First Spontaneous Vaginal Delivery," *The Journal of Obstetrics & Gynecology*. 96(2): 214–18, Aug. 2000.

4. *biotech.law.lsu.edu*

Chapter 10 — *Breastfeeding*

1. D.C. Brown, "Smoking cessation in pregnancy," *Can Fam Physician 1996*; 42:102–5 [review]

Chapter 12 — *CIMS*

1. Mother-Friendly Childbirth Initiative from the Coalition for Improving Maternity Services (CIMS), www.motherfriendly.org.
   Email: info@motherfriendly.org,
   P.O. Box 2346, Ponte Vedra Beach, FL 32004, 1-888-282-2467

2. World Health Organization: WHO is governed by 192 member-states through the World Health Assembly, which is composed of representatives from WHO's member-states. The main tasks of the World Health Assembly are to approve the WHO program and the budget for the following biennium and to decide major policy questions.

3. A. Langer, et al., "Effects of psychosocial support during labor and childbirth on breastfeeding, medical interventions, and mother's wellbeing in a Mexican public hospital: A randomized clinical trial," *British Journal of Obstetrics and Gynecology*, 105, 10561063, 1988

   U. Waldenstrom, and D. Turnbull, "A systematic review comparing continuity of midwifery care with standard maternity services," *British Journal of Obstetrics and Gynecology*, 105, 11601170, 1998

   G. Berkowitz, K. Scott, and M. Klaus, "A comparison of intermittent and continuous support during labor: A meta-analysis," *American Journal of Obstetrics and Gynecology*, 180 (5), 10541059, 1999

   B. C. Madi, et al., "Effects of female relative support in labor: A randomized controlled trial," *Birth*, 26 (1), 48, 1999

4. ibid.

5. K. Gaffney, et al., "Stressful events among pregnant Salvadoran women: A cross-cultural comparison," *Journal of Obstetric, Gynecological, and Neonatal Nursing,* 26 (3), 303310, 1997

    J. Howard, and V. Berbiglia, "Caring for childbearing Korean women," *Journal of Obstetric, Gynecological, and Neonatal Nursing,* 26 (6), 665671, 1997

    S. Weber, "Cultural aspects of pain in childbearing women," *Journal of Obstetric, Gynecological, and Neonatal Nursing,* 25 (1), 6772, 1996

    M. Sweeney, and C. Guilino, "The health belief model as an explanation for breastfeeding practices in Hispanic population," *Advanced Nursing Science,* 9 (4), 3550, 1987

6. M. Rossi, and S. Lindell, "Maternal positions and pushing techniques in a nonprescriptive environment," *Journal of Obstetric, Gynecological and Neonatal Nursing* (15), 203208, 1986

    L. Albers, et al., "The relationship of ambulation in labor to operative delivery," *The Journal of Nurse-Midwifery,* 42(1), 48, 1997

7. S. Godman Brown, and B. Tate Johnson, "Enhancing early discharge with home follow-up: A pilot project," *Journal of Obstetric, Gynecological, and Neonatal Nursing,* 27 (1), 3338, 1998

    V. Mendler, et al., "The conception, birth, and infancy of an early discharge program," *American Journal of Maternal Child Nursing,* 21, 241246, 1996

8. L. Albers, and D. Savitz, "Hospital setting for birth and use of medical procedures in low-risk women" (abstract), *Journal of Nurse Midwifery,* 36(6)

    J. Rooks, N. Weatherby, and E. Y Ernst, "The National Birth Center Study Part II: Intrapartum and immediate postpartum and neonatal care" (abstract), *Journal of Nurse Midwifery,* 37(5), 301330, 1992

    M. L. Romney, and H. Gordon, "Is your enema really necessary?" (abstract), *British Medical Journal,* 282(6272), 12691271, 1981

    S. Drayton, and C. Rees, "They know what they are doing" (abstract), *Nursing Mirror,* 159(5), 48, 1984

N. Johnson, et al., "Randomized trial comparing a policy of early with selective amniotomy in uncomplicated labour at term" (abstract), *British Journal of Obstetrics and Gynaecology*, 104, 340346, 1997

J. Barrett, et al., "Randomized trial of amniotomy in labour versus the intention to leave membranes intact until the second stage" (abstract), *British Journal of Obstetrics and Gynaecology*, 99, 59, 1992

F. Goffinet, et al., "Early amniotomy increases the frequency of fetal heart rate abnormalities" (abstract), *British Journal of Obstetrics and Gynaecology*, 104, 548553, 1997

Bansal, K. R. et al., "Is there a benefit to episiotomy at spontaneous vaginal delivery? A natural experiment" (abstract), American Journal of Obstetrics and Gynecology, 175(4), 897901, 1996

Signorello, L. B. et al., "Midline episiotomy and anal incontinence: Retrospective cohort study" (abstract), British Medical Journal, 320, 8790, 2000

Goyert, G. et al., "The physician factor in cesarean birth rates" (abstract), New England Journal of Medicine, 320(11), 706709, 1989

Hemminki, E. and Merilainen, J., "Long-term effects of cesarean sections: Ectopic pregnancies and placental problems" (abstract), American Journal of Obstetrics and Gynecology, 174(5), 15691574, 1996

9. Rush, J. et al., "The effects of whirlpool baths in labor: A randomized, controlled trial" (abstract), Birth, 23, 136143, 1996

Wiand, N. E., "Relaxation levels achieved by Lamaze-trained pregnant women listening to music and ocean sound tapes" (abstract), *The Journal of Perinatal Education*, 6(4), 18, 1997

E. Burns, and C. Blamey, "Using aromatherapy in childbirth" (abstract), *Nursing Times*, 90(9), 54, 56, 58, 1994

B. H. McCrea, and M.E. Wright, "Satisfaction in childbirth and perceptions of personal control in pain relief during labour" (abstract), *Journal of Advanced Nursing*, 29(4), 877884, 1999

10. ibid.

11. B. Stevens, C. Johnston, R. and Grunan, "Issues of assessment of pain and discomfort in neonates" (abstract), *Journal of Obstetric, Gynecologic and Neonatal Nursing,* 24(9), 849855, 1995

F. Porter, C. Wolf, and J. P. Miller, "Procedural pain in newborn infants: The influence of intensity and development" (abstract), *Pediatrics,* 104(1), e13, 1999

J. Lawrence, et al., "The development of a tool to assess neonatal pain" (abstract), *Neonatal Network,* 12(6), 5966, 1993

T. To, et al., "Cohort study on circumcision of newborn boys and subsequent risk of urinary-tract infection" (abstract), *Journal of Urology,* 162(4), 1562, 1999, and additional articles that support non-circumcision (not abstracted)

Index

NOTES

NOTES

NOTES

NOTES

NOTES

NOTES

NOTES

NOTES

NOTES

NOTES

NOTES

NOTES

NOTES